W0227934

Interpersonal
Psychiatry

Interpersonal Psychiatry

Patrick Mullahy, M.A.
Associate Professor Emeritus of Psychology
Manhattan College, New York

and

Menachem Melinek, M.D.
Associate Director of Psychiatry
The Bronx Lebanon Hospital Center
and
Assistant Professor of Psychiatry
Albert Einstein College of Medicine
New York

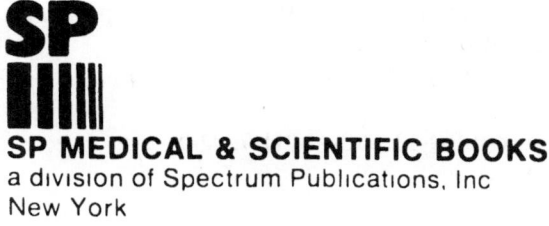

SP MEDICAL & SCIENTIFIC BOOKS
a division of Spectrum Publications, Inc
New York

Copyright © 1983 by Spectrum Publications, Inc.

Softcover reprint of the hardcover 1st edition 1983

All rights reserved. No part of this book may be reproduced in any form, by photostat, microform, retrieval system, or any other means without prior written permission of the copyright holder or his licensee.

SPECTRUM PUBLICATIONS, INC.
175-20 Wexford Terrace
Jamaica, NY 11432

Library of Congress Cataloging in Publication Data

Mullahy, Patrick, 1912–
   Interpersonal psychiatry.

   Bibliography: p.
   Includes index.
   1. Sullivan, Harry Stack, 1892–1949. 2. Psychoanalysis.
3. Interpersonal relations. 4. Child psychology. 5. Psychology,
Pathological. I. Melinek, Menachem. II. Title. [DNLM: 1. Interpersonal
relations. 2. Mental disorders. WM 100 M955i]
RC339.52.S87M84   1983   616.89′092′4   82-23045

ISBN-13: 978-94-011-7294-3   e-ISBN-13: 978-94-011-7292-9
DOI: 10.1007/ 978-94-011-7292-9

Publisher's Note

This volume represents both triumph and tragedy. We believe this to be a landmark contribution to the field of human behavior; a reinterpretation of one of the giants of psychiatry by an internationally acclaimed interpreter who with the collaboration of a younger colleague has now brought us to an even greater appreciation of the theories of Henry Stack Sullivan.

Tragically, neither author has lived to see this work published. We, therefore, sadly dedicate this book to their memory and to their respective families.

In Memoriam

Patrick F. Mullahy was born in County Mayo, Ireland in February of 1912 and emigrated to the United States in 1927. He worked his way through City College of New York and did his graduate work at Columbia University in philosophy. He became a close friend of Harry Stack Sullivan and developed a very strong interest in psychology. His first book, *Oedipus Myth and Complex*, published in 1948, was acclaimed nationally and internationally. In addition to numerous journal articles, he edited *A Study of Interpersonal Relations* (1949) and *The Contributions of Harry Stack Sullivan* (1952). He also wrote the section on Sullivan for *The Comprehensive Textbook of Psychiatry*. He taught at Hunter College of the City University of New York during the 1950's and in the early 1960's began teaching at Manhattan College in Riverdale, New York. In 1970, he published his most important work on Sullivan, *Psychoanalysis and Interpersonal Psychiatry*. He died on September 13, 1982, of heart failure shortly after the completion of this present work.

My thanks to Dr. Maurice Green for his help and advice to my father during the writing of this book. In addition, I would like to express appreciation to my aunt, Mrs. Ann O'Neill (Mullahy) for her love and attention to my father throughout his life and for her help with this foreword.

PATRICIA MULLAHY

Menacham Melinek was a friend and colleague. He was Associate Director of Psychiatry at the Bronx-Lebanon Hospital Center, and Assistant Professor of Psychiatry at the Albert Einstein College of Medicine. The last major endeavor he completed before his untimely death was working with Patrick Mullahy in writing and updating Mullahy's classic book on Interpersonal Psychiatry. This book is a tribute to the knowledge, wisdom, and maturity of Dr. Mullahy, and to the energy and resourcefulness of Dr. Melinek. Dr. Melinek's death was not only an irreparable loss to his family and friends but to his profession as well.

HARVEY BLUESTONE, MD

Preface

An impressive amount of work, experimental, statistical and "observational" or "phenomenological" has been done in psychiatry during the past 30 to 40 years. Although Sullivan's achievements have placed him in the first rank of psychiatry, some of the work done since he died in 1949 can be assimilated to enchance his achievements. For this reason, I enlisted the aid of Menachem Melinek, M.D., whose wide knowledge of recent and contemporary psychiatric studies is admirably suited to the task of assimilating some of them to Sullivan's theories.

PATRICK MULLAHY

Preface

Acknowledgments

The authors wish to acknowledge with gratitude Mrs. Mari Hughes, formerly secretary, Department of Psychology, Manhattan College, for typing the original manuscript. Dr. Robert G. Kvarnes of the Washington School of Psychiatry, read the original manuscript and contributed several keen criticisms and suggestions for which we are grateful.

We wish to express our thanks to the Department of Psychiatry, at Montefiore-North Central Bronx Hospitals for the support in preparing the final manuscript of the book. Robert Steinmuller, Director of Psychiatry at North Central Bronx Hospital was generous with his help. We would like as well to acknowledge the support of the Department of Psychiatry at Bronx-Lebanon Hospital Center and its Director of Psychiatry, Dr. Harvey Bluestone.

PATRICK MULLAHY
MENACHEM MELINEK

Contents

Contents

Interpersonal
Psychiatry

Sullivan and Freud

INTRODUCTION

The purpose of this book is to expound the more fundamental ideas of Harry Stack Sullivan's psychology in order to provide the reader with a broad grasp of the "theory" of interpersonal psychiatry and to supplement it with certain recent developments. Like every other creative thinker, Sullivan learned much from his predecessors and, in certain instances, his contemporaries as well. Recently, Sullivan's debt to the late Adolf Meyer, of Johns Hopkins University, particularly in regard to Sullivan's ideas about about schizophrenia, has been emphasized. In addition, Adlerians would be critical if Alfred Adler's contributions to Sullivan's psychology were not mentioned. Adler possessed a profound grasp of the individual in community, and, in a sense, was an interpersonal theorist, at least in his work with patients. But in general, Adler's individual psychology is profoundly different from Sullivan's (Cooley, 1962). However, Henri F. Ellenberger (1970) in his *The Discovery of the Unconscious* has done ample justice to Adler. It can be said that the man to whom Sullivan was most indebted was Sigmund Freud. Sullivan began his career attempting to follow strictly the psychiatry of Freud. But, in his work with schizophrenic patients, classical psychoanalysis was quite inadequate. So, Sullivan began his lifelong attempt to construct more adequate modalities of treatment for those patients who did not seem to benefit from a strict psychoanalytic approach. Thus, a visitor to an inpatient psychiatric ward of a facility today would be struck by the enormous influence of Sullivan's contribution, as manifested in the commonly used milieu therapy. The extensive summary of Freudian theory in this chapter is meant to provide an illuminating perspective with the help of which, it is hoped, the reader can achieve a broader point of view of the interpersonal school of psychiatry. For Sullivan, Freud served as a foil against whom he developed his own "theories."

Leston L. Havens (1973) in his book *Approaches to the Mind* has recently appraised Sullivan as follows:

"Harry Stack Sullivan is the most original figure in American psychiatry, the only American to help found a major school. He stares past us now, two decades after his death, through those nearsighted Joycean Irish eyes, half participating and half observing, his own man to the last. We will have to answer the high European contempt for his *psychiatrie de concierge* to take full pride in him, but pride we should take in this great American contributor to the mainstream of psychiatric advance."

Kraepelin, one of the first categorizers of modern psychiatry, conceived of mental or psychological processes as occurring within an encapsulated psyche. Meyer and Sullivan should be credited for the movement outward from this tradition. In Chapter 3 of Freud's *New Introductory Lectures on Psychoanalysis*, (Freud, 1949) "The Anatomy of the Mental Personality," one can obtain a rapid glimpse of his conception of the mind as self-enclosed, more or less self-actional. Yet, as Havens (1973) points out, Freudian psychopathology is everywhere shot through with considerations of social factors "despite Freud's fundamental bias, so heavily shared with Kraepelin, for intra-individual concepts such as instincts and energies." Man is a social being and no one can ignore it. For Sullivan the "intra-psychic" is always a part or sub-category of an interpersonal configuration. Experience is the inner component of events in which a living organism participates as such—that is, as an organized entity.

Freud's Mental Topography

For Freud, psychic processes occur within three more or less interrelated psychological systems—Id, Ego and Superego. The three may work harmoniously, or painful conflicts may arise, such as that between the Ego and Superego. According to Sullivan, personality embodies the Self (which can be crudely and superficially translated into the Superego and Ego) and the Dissociated (which can be crudely and superficially translated into the unconscious—Id).

In light of what has already been said, it is not difficult to understand that the main unit of study for Freud is the more or less self-contained individual. For Sullivan, the unit of study is always an interpersonal situation or an ongoing series of interpersonal processes.

Freud's Formulation of Instincts

Leaving aside Freud's last formulation of instincts briefly, one can point out that during a period of many years he asserted that human life is governed by two classes of more or less fixed drives or CR instincts.

(These should not be confused with reflexes). These are the instincts of self-preservation (the ego instincts) and the instincts of racial preservation (the sexual instincts). In contrast, Sullivan did not formulate his conceptions within the framework of instincts.

An instinct, according to Freud, may be characterized by having (1) a source of excitation within the body; (2) an *aim*, i.e., the removal of that excitation; and (3) an *object*, the means by which and toward which an aim is ordinarily directed and its achievement accomplished or fulfilled. It also has an *impetus*, strength or force.

Freud wrote that satisfaction of the aim can often be achieved in the subject's own body by some kind of somatic modification; although usually, an external object is introduced in which and by which the instinct achieves its aim. The sexual aims of individuals during infancy and early childhood are often achieved "in their own body." Of course, in adult life, an external sexual object, to use Freud's language, is normally introduced. There is one thing that needs to be mentioned in connection with the Freudian formulation of instincts. Sullivan did not conceive such a rigid dichotomy of inner and outer. For the latter, an eternal commerce (transaction) is occurring between the person who possesses various needs, somatic and psychic, and the outer world, both physical and social.

THE THEORY OF INSTINCTS

A "theory" of instincts plays a fundamental role in Freudian psychology. But, although it is a basal conception or set of conceptions, Freud asserts it is obscure and conventional (at least it was conventional 50 or 60 years ago). The conception of instinct may have been partly derived from physiology. Freud wrote that physiology has given us the concept of stimuli and the scheme of the reflex arc, according to which a stimulus coming from the outer world and processed in the nervous system is discharged by action toward the outer world. Among other things, this action serves the purpose of withdrawal, an overt event removing it from the operation of the stimulus or event. A very simple example is that of a light striking the eye, which acts as such a stimulus, effecting a characteristic response such as blinking. But, a complex stimulus such as hunger, sets off a chain of conditioned responses arousing the feeding process.

There are other stimuli which come from within the organism. The internal stimulus is said by Freud to be, in several vital respects, quite different from the external. It never acts as a momentary impact, but as a *constant force;* it is inescapable. One can usually flee from noxious or powerful external stimuli, but one cannot escape hunger or thirst without satisfaction. And, although sexual stimuli may be—and seemingly are—of a different order from hunger or thirst, a healthy individual cannot rid himself of them by overt physical activity. In any event, the internal stimulus is said to be instinctual.

Freud pictured an instinct as a certain sum or quantity of energy forcing its way in a certain direction. He wrote that from a biological point of view, an instinct appears as a borderline concept, between the mental and the physical. An instinct is both the mental representative of the stimuli emanating from within the organism and penetrating to the mind, and at the same time, a measure of the demand made upon the psyche, in consequence of its connection with the body. For example, the sexual instinct's mental representation in an adult appears in the form of a certain quality of feeling, which *up to a certain level of intensity,* can be exquisitely pleasurable, and is recognized as sexual excitement emanating from the genital zone. At the same time, the intensity of the feeling or excitement may be a measure or indication of the effort required by the mind or psyche to relieve the excitement by appropriate sexual activity. Presumably, the greater the instinctual stimulus, as manifested by feeling, the greater will be the energy required to relieve it. However, some people have weak sexual drives and seem to get along comfortably without any apparent sexual activity. Biologically, sex "presses for fulfillment," Salzman (1962) has written,

> with no greater urgency than hunger, thirst, or other basic physiological need. It can, as a matter of fact, be more easily abandoned than any other physiological need. This is demonstrated in the life of the ascetic or in religious movements. In circumstances of deprivation, it can be easily abandoned....In addition, most individuals will cling tenaciously to certain ideals or values, relinquishing sexual satisfactions for long periods of time if necessary.

(Whether this is as true during the periods of decline of civilizations, however, is not so certain.) Ruch and Zimbardo (1971) present an excellent brief analysis of the sexual drive, its meaning and manifestations in man and animal which might be found useful.

Freud's notion that powerful sexual instincts can be sublimated during adolescence is open to question, especially if one lacks a rigorous moral code. Sullivan did not try to explain all these complex phenomena by one ego function, e.g. sublimation. He thought that art, for example, is inexplicable, and he did not accept the simple explanation of Freud. There is another point that one needs to be wary of with reference to Freud. Other powerful drives, such as loneliness, aggressiveness, and the desire for status can be unconsciously "displaced," or disguised, and appear in consciousness as sexual attraction toward someone or a lingering sexual interest.

THE NEW THEORY OF INSTINCTS

For certain somewhat complicated reasons, Freud revised his conceptions of the instincts around 1920 (Ellenberger, 1970). These conceptions are labeled Thanatos (Death Instinct) or Self-Destructive Instinct, and Eros or Life-Furthering Instinct. The new formulation made its appearance in *Beyond the Pleasure Principle*, published in 1920. Hitherto, the Pleasure Principle, which may be characterized as the desire to achieve a maximum amount of pleasure under the given circumstances of life, while avoiding as much pain or *unpleasure (unlust)* as possible. But, the Death Instinct is more fundamental; it has "overthrown" the Pleasure Principle. The goal of life is death because, as Ellenberger (1970) says, the preservation instinct or Ego Instinct is one aspect of the death instinct, since it protects against accidental, externally caused death, in order to preserve the individual for death from internal causes.

Further caution is needed here. Someone who is versed in biology or biochemistry may get the impression that Freud is writing about the as yet more or less obscure chemistry of the living cell, which is born and for unknown or partially unknown causes runs its course and dies. However, the contemporary knowledge of biology and chemistry did not exist in 1920. Ellenberger seems to suggest Freud may have been influenced by the philosopher Schopenhauer. The more likely explanation is that Freud lived the major part of his professional life during what has been called the most evil century in history, the twentieth. Of course, this is no proof of the existence of a Death Instinct. Nor is it a valid explanation for the occurrence of wars, irrational social movements and genocide as Freudians used to believe.

By and large, the previous formulation of the Ego Instincts and Sexual Instincts were subsumed in Freud's new theory under Eros, and a new formulation of the Instincts added, the Destructive Instincts whose aim was destruction—often of others if it seems feasible, but, in any case, ultimately oneself. The energy at the disposal of Eros is libidinal energy. But, curiously enough, Freud either overlooked, or was unable to speculate on, what the energy at the disposal of the Destructive Instincts was. These two kinds of instincts are inherent in every particle of living matter. The association and opposition of these two forces create the phenomena of life. Eros and Thanatos may combine and fuse (or draw apart) so that the destructive power of Thanatos is temporarily allayed, but it eventually triumphs. In a very unclear fashion, Freud thought that these forces were constituents of living cells and their combination — a problem he briefly touches upon in *Beyond the Pleasure Principle*. Sullivan regarded these ideas as having dubious validity and probably destructive for therapeutic purposes because they force the therapist to search for a psychology of the person that does not exist.

The Rigidity of Freud's Instinct Conceptions

It should now be clear that Freud's instincts, in the light of contemporary psychology, are too fixed, and too rigidly conceived (Sartain et al., 1973). It is fair to say that his psychology is essentially based on a biological model, however inadequate. One should remember that Freud grew to manhood during the heyday of Darwinian biology, with its emphasis on instincts. (See Ruch and Zimbardo [1971] for example, for a summary of the contemporary conceptions of instinct.)

Freud's Conceptions of the Ego

It is inaccurate to write that Freud held this or that "theory" of personality development; he never constructed any. His ideas on the *development* of the ego can be summed up briefly. Even when he had created a theory of personality "organization," he still maintained that the ego is "weak," since it has no energy of its own and borrows it from the Id. Furthermore, the ego has to serve three harsh masters: the Superego, the Id and Reality, when it has reached the development of the adolescent or adult, or somewhat sooner, depending on one's level of maturity.

The description of the emergence of the Ego out of the Id is cursory, as previously mentioned. In *An Outline of Psychoanalysis* Freud (1949) wrote:

> Under the influence of the external world which surrounds us, one portion of the Id has undergone a special development. From what was originallly a cortical layer, provided with organs for receiving stimuli and with apparatus for protection against excessive stimulation, a special organization has arisen which henceforward acts as an intermediary between the Id and the external world. This region of our mental life has been given the name of Ego.

It should be remembered that the nervous system, from a biological standpoint, ultimately controls the action of our muscles and glands, as well as being an instrumentality of sensation, perception, and thought. The latter three deal with consciousness. Perhaps these phenomena are more interrelated than have been mentioned. For example, there is a close relationship between the activities of the brain and those of the sense organs, but that is of little significance for our purposes. There seems to be no way of reconciling the action of the nervous system, which is a physical system, and consciousness, which is part of the psyche and evolves gradually except by an analysis that is foreign to Freud's thought. Although one should not become sidetracked by philosophical discussion, Abraham Edel's book, *The Theory and Practice of Philosophy* (Edel, 1946) is recommended.

In his description of the Ego's functions, Freud added that, in consequence of the relation which was already established between (the nervous system) sensory perception and muscular action, the Ego is in control of voluntary action. But, it has many other functions, including self-preservation, awareness of the external world, storing up experiences in the memory, avoiding excessive stimuli, and learning through activity in order to bring about appropriate modifications in the external world.

The second great task of the Ego, which often proves difficult, deals with *internal* events, in relation to the Id. The latter is the ultimate source of the instincts, which are connected with bodily needs and demands, giving them mental representation. The Ego maintains control of the instincts, (which are of themselves blind) as best it can by gaining control over their imperious demands, be deciding whether they shall be allowed to obtain satisfaction, by postponing satisfactions to times and circumstances favorable in the external world, or by suppressing (and repressing) their excitations completely.

Summarily, the activities of the Ego are said to be governed by consideration of the tensions produced by stimuli present within it or introduced into it. Freud wrote that the raising of these tensions to an unspecified level is in general felt as *unpleasure* and their lowering as *pleasurable*. The demands and requirements of bodily, mental, and environmental interrelationships govern levels of tension. Id, Ego, and Superego are foreign to Sullivan's formulations. Where Freud talks about Ego and Superego, Sullivan talks about the Self System (anti-anxiety system) and the Dissociated system. It could be said that the self system experiences as well as acts, with reference to personality. The dissociated system is brought into light only under certain circumstances of interpersonal relations; but it too is an aspect of personality.

The Character of Tension

Tension is a conception that has aroused a great deal of controversy caused perhaps by misunderstanding. "It is probable, however," Freud wrote, "that what is felt as *pleasure* and *unpleasure* is not the *absolute* degree of the tensions, but something in the rhythm of their changes" (Freud, 1949). Although Ego seeks pleasure and seeks to avoid unpleasure, the physiological substrate is a rhythm of change, not a comatose quiescence. This idea is in harmony with commonsense experience. An increase in unpleasure which is expected and foreseen is said to be met by a signal of anxiety, the occasion of which is danger from without or within (the Id). Sullivan's approach to anxiety tension was that it was the expression of the lowering self esteem. More generally, for Sullivan, tension is a potentiality for action, or the transformation of energy in the various activities of life.

More or less periodically, the Ego abandons its connection with the world and withdraws into *sleep*, a study of which Freud made in his *Interpretation of Dreams* (Luce, 1966). During the state of sleep, the organization of the Ego undergoes far-reaching changes, some of which approach a schizophrenia-like state (primary processes) as nightmares. Nevertheless, in a deep, dreamless sleep, the psyche undergoes a minimum of stimulation. In sleep, the Ego temporarily withdraws from the world. It can and does revert to a more primitive level, free of the work-a-day world, at least in normal people. For Freud, during sleep, dreams provided the key to an understanding of mental life. Sullivan, it can be said, put much less stress on dreams; although he employed them in his therapeutic approach at times. Although he did not profess to have a theory of dreams, Sullivan claimed that Freud's ideas about latent dream content were unverifiable. The therapist is always limited to what he can learn from the manifest dream or dream fragments.

Defense Mechanisms

Since the Ego's task is chiefly self-preservation and self esteem, as previously characterized, it has another quite distinctive set of functions called *defense mechanisms* (in Sullivan's terms, "security operations"), which help to ward off or alleviate conflicts and anxieties. It should be noted that defense mechanisms always operate unconsciously. They include mechanisms such as rationalization, repression, regression, projection, and sublimation. Although they have been variously formulated, only their essential meanings will be elaborated here.

Rationalization

To *rationalize* is to offer a more or less plausible but pseudo explanation, to oneself or to others, as circumstances warrant, for something one thinks, says, or does and which would otherwise cause anxiety and conflict. The term was first used by the English psychoanalyst, Ernest Jones, in 1908, whose chief claim to fame is perhaps that he wrote an official biography of Freud.

Repression

In Freudian psychology, *repression* has two related meanings: (a) confining id-impulses which are constantly striving for an outlet within the boundaries of the Id; and (b) forcing back into the Id any impulse that has escaped its boundaries which is intolerable to the Ego because of its values and beliefs or because any overt expression of such an impulse in the external world could be dangerous if it conflicts with the folkways, mores, and laws of the community. Sullivan also thought that what Freud called repression ("dissociation") might be involved in any intense anxiety provoking course of events. But, he employed "selective inattention" more frequently as an instrumentality of the self.

Regression

Regression means either (a) reverting to the sort of objects, parents or their surrogates, to which one was attached as a child; or (b) a reversion of the entire psychic apparatus — the entire personality — to the sort of organization and functions characteristic of it at an earlier stage. In either sense, regression occurs when one encounters some crisis or problem which cannot be resolved. Some event or situation occurs which is too painful, dangerous, or anxiety-provoking to be borne. Freud often discovered that his patients had suffered an incipient "neurosis" during the course of childhood so that, at least to a degree, their libidinal development was halted or arrested during this phase; an occurrence which Freud called a *fixation point*. It is to this fixation point that neurotic patients revert. Of course, a similar fate occurs to the ego, but Freud does not stress it. Sullivan did not theoretically elaborate much on the mechanism of regression. It was a return to or a reactivation of some earlier phase of development or some earlier occurrences. Sullivan addressed himself to fixation and called it an arrest of development, This will be discussed subsequently.

Projection

In *projection* one attributes (unconsciously, of course) to some other person or group some characteristic or set of characteristics which he unknowingly possesses, characteristics that he regards as obnoxious or intolerable because of his values and beliefs. Sullivan essentially agreed with Freud's formulation of projection, although, having suggested that the degree to which people with chronically low self-esteem anticipate unfavorable opinions in others, he proceeded to state that he did not think that "the mechanism of projection accounts for much of anything" (Sullivan, 1953). Projection is chiefly distorted misperception often evoked by anxiety.

Sublimation

As a defense mechanism *sublimation* is troublesome to formulate. One thing it is *not:* the conscious rechanneling of one's energies toward the achievement of new goals. The rechanneling is an unconscious process, directed towad the achievement of higher ends — social, artistic, scientific, or philosophic. Sublimation implies, firstly, that one has some threatening impulse — threatening because its overt expression in the real world could be dangerous or unwise or; secondly, threatening to one's own Ego with its configuration of values and beliefs. Although

Freud does not seem to make it very clear, when sublimation occurs, the energy which one employs undergoes a qualitative change. He employs sublimation chiefly in relation to the sexual and destructive instincts. Given his very pessimistic appraisal of man's nature, it is not surprising that he thought civilization was built up at the cost of sexual and aggressive instincts. That is to say, without the repression and sublimation of man's primitive, primordial instincts, civilization would never have developed. This matter is discussed at length in Freud's *Civilization and Its Discontents*, in which he provides a very unlovely picture of human nature. For Sullivan, creativity is inexplicable; no one can explain its nature. Therefore, to say that the creative work of art and science is a sublimation of this or that tells nothing.

Distinctive Qualities of Awareness

Before turning to a discussion of the Superego, it is important that the psyche is characterized by three characteristics: conscious, preconscious, and unconscious qualities. In various writings, previous to roughly 1920, Freud had formulated the three qualities of awareness, consciousness, preconsciousness and unconsciousness as "psychic regions" or "mental localities." This is an illustration of the fact that Freud's extensive use of metaphor often disguised the obscurity of some of his ideas. In any case, among his later writings, consciousness is taken to be a self-evident quality of the mind, a fact which one would have to assume in every attempt to "explain" it. Of course, consciousness depends on a functioning organism in which the nervous system plays a vital role, but it is no more synonymous with the workings of the nervous system than is the soul of Christian philosophy. Unfortunately, simplistic explanations have been offered for matters that baffle the most brilliant minds. In any case, we begin with consciousness, as William James used to write, as a primitive postulate: We accept it as surely as we take for granted the existence of oxygen in the atmosphere. Still, one must admit that Freud attached more efficacy to the unconscious part of the mind. In this sense, Freud was a supreme irrationalist who contributed his share to the decline of faith in reason.

> At first we might be inclined to think very much less of the importance of consciousness as a criterion (of reality), since it has proved so unworthy. But if we did so, we should be wrong. It is the same with life: it is not worth much but it is all we have (Freud, 1949).

Preconsciousness pertains to what is temporarily unconscious. Normally, we pay little attention to it, taking it for granted as we do consciousness. Yet, almost all the knowledge and experience we can recall and recollect is ordinarily preconscious.

Unconsciousness has a *definite*, although not always clear, meaning for Freud. In various contexts, it may be regarded as a characteristic or manifestation of the Id. When applied to the Ego or Superego, it is purely descriptive; that is, it is not a system in Freud's latest formulations, although in *A General Introduction to Psychoanalysis* (Freud, 1943) and elsewhere, it is. The unconsciousness of the Id has a very different quality from that of consciousness or preconsciousness, or even the unconsciousness of the Ego or Superego. In the Id, unconsciousness is essential, since the Id is entirely unconscious. The two are always inseparable. In *An Outline of Psychoanalysis* Freud (1949) wrote that the sole quality that rules in the Id is that of being unconscious and irrational. He added that the Id and unconscious are as intimately united as Ego and preconscious; that the former connection is even more exclusive. The unconsciousness of the Id is of a more primitive quality of awareness. In everyday life, we know nothing about it, although it manifests itself obscurely in dreams, slips of the tongue or of the pen, and in various other phenomena of everyday life. What Freud called infantile amnesia is due, in part, to this property of the mind. For example, a teacher may be impressed by how little college students seem able to remember of their lives before they started school. Infantile amnesia is a rich source of study though it transcends the scope of this book (See Schachtel, 1959).

In *Personal Psychopathology* Sullivan (1972) wrote:

> Dissociation is a process by which some of the systems of experience and some of the somatic apparatus are disintegrated from the rest of the personality and engaged in overt and implicit quasi adjustive processes not in harmony with those of the rest of the personality.

Dissociation is the outcome of intense disapproval by parents and others so that the anxiety when experienced, perhaps as early as late infancy, gives rise to a bifurcation of experience. Hence, from very early in life there is a split in the development of personality. Dissociated experiences become foreign to the experiences of the growing self. Eventually, the personality becomes constituted of two "systems," each foreign to the other. These ideas are more or less parallel to the early Freudian ideas of the unconscious psychic apparatus.

THE SUPEREGO

Although Freud's conceptions of the Superego were briefly discussed, they will be elaborated on at this point. The Freudian Superego is very rigorous and harsh in its demands on, and regulation of, the Ego. Some have ascribed these characteristics of the Superego to Freud's Jewish origins; others to his having grown to manhood during the Victorian Era, (concerning which many of us have many false ideas). Nevertheless, Freud's world was very different from the current one. It seems doubtful that most Americans now harbor a conscience as rigorous and severe as the Superego Freud attributed to the denizens of Middle Europe he knew in the early part of this century. In fact, many readers, for example, in the United States regard traditional morality with disdain or indifference. Some seem to equate morality with sexual morality, which would be traditional morality, they say, if they accepted it to limit their freedom. Others regard traditional morality, in general, as spurious and a hindrance to their self-fulfillment. They have their own morality, they say, although as a rule it is difficult to discover what it is. Whether any society can long survive without a generally shared and strongly held set of moral beliefs is open to question, although we must pass it by (Green, 1952).

In his *Outline of Psychoanalysis* Freud (1949) wrote:

> The long period of childhood during which the growing human being lives in dependence upon his parents, leaves behind it a precipitate which forms within his Ego a special agency in which this parental influence is prolonged.

In this last of his published works, Freud seems to attribute more importance to the mother than in previous works, where the significance of the father in the formation of the Superego is paramount. But, the actual difference, if any, is slight. The parents' natural influence is said to include not merely the personalities of the parents themselves, but also the racial, national, and familial traditions handed on through them, as well as the demands of the immediate social milieu which they represent. Additionally, an individual's Superego may, in the course of his development, adopt contributions from successors to his parents, such as teachers, admired figures in public life, or high social ideals. To adopt a subjective morality is to have no morality.

Curiously, Freud thought that the Superego seems to have made a one-sided selection and to have chosen only the harshness and severity of the parents—their preventive and punitive functions. Even when they have reared the child with gentleness and kindness and have avoided threats of punishment insofar as possible, the Superego reflects the same relentless harshness as if the parents had ruled with a rod of iron. But this seeming paradox is explained by Freud's conception that the Superego receives its energy from the Id, which lends the former its cruel, sadistic characteristics and activities.

The Superego is often translated as *conscience*, but it is different from the traditional Christian notion of conscience. The Superego is primarily a reflection of conventional mores, of the conventional "shoulds" and "should nots" of a given society, while in the traditional Christian view conscience reflects universal, objective moral norms.

The Superego has another aspect: the ego ideal, by which one measures oneself; a vision of the good toward which one strives, and whose demands for ever-increasing perfection one is always striving to fulfill. But for Freud, there is no innate striving for the ideal. He regarded the ideal as a "recipitation" or residue of the *old* idea of the parents, when as a young child one regarded them as splendid, almost god-like figures, expressing the admiration which the young child felt for them and which he gradually modified as he grew older. It is very instructive to compare the ego-ideal envisioned by William James, a generation earlier, in his *Principles of Psychology* (1907), with that of Freud. The lyrical exposition of that great seminal thinker (a phrase of Alfred North Whitehead) is in marked contrast to Freud's conception of the ego-ideal. Instead of writing of Superego, Sullivan wrote about the supervisory patterns of the self. These include various "critics" such as the "Hearer," the "Spectator," the "Writing Critic," etc. All these will be discussed in a later chapter. There is no such thing as an ego ideal in Sullivan's theory, at least explicitly, but compare his *Psychiatric Interview* where the germ of an ego-idea may be formed.

THE ID (UNCONSCIOUS PSYCHICAL SYSTEM)

Freud explained that psychoanalytic work compelled him to use the word *unconscious* in more than one sense. For example, he discovered, he wrote, that large and important regions of the mind are normally removed from knowledge of the Ego, so that the processes which occur in them must be recognized as unconscious in the true dynamic sense of the term. That is, he attributed a topographical or systemic meaning to the word *unconscious*. In other words, the unconscious was conceived as a psychical system. For such reasons, Freud revised his formulations of the anatomy of the personality. The Unconscious as a System was replaced by the term Id. The other two systems are Ego and Superego. Ego and Superego are to a considerable extent unconscious; they exist and operate unconsciously only in a "descriptive" sense, that is, as levels of awareness. The Id is unconscious; it has no preconscious or conscious characteristics or attributes. The primitive intellectual processes characteristic of dreams occur in the Id. If we were to examine these matters in detail, we might discover our distinctions are not so entirely clear-cut, but that would transcend the purpose of this book.

The oldest of the three mental provinces is the Id. It is said to contain everything that is inherited, present at birth, and fixed in the constitution. The instincts which originate in the somatic organization acquire their first mental representation in the Id. Freud wrote that the Id is the obscure, inaccessible part of the personality. The little he learned about it, he claimed, he learned from the study and interpretation of dreams (which, in a disguised form, express the contents of the Id), as well as from the formation of neurotic symptoms. The Id may be pictured as "a chaos, a cauldron, of seething excitement" (Freud, 1949). The Id is in direct contact with somatic processes and takes over from them instinctual needs, giving them mental expression but, the substratum where the contact is made, is unknown.

> These instincts fill it with energy, but it has no organization and no unified will, only an impulsion to obtain satisfaction for the instinctual needs in accordance with the Pleasure Principle (Freud, 1949).

Processes in the Id know no laws of logic, especially the principle of contradiction, since contradictory impulses can exist side by side. Negation of any sort is unknown to it. Since there is nothing in the Id corresponding to the recognition of the passage of time, no alteration of impulses occurs through time.

> Conative impulses which have never gotten beyond the Id, and even impressions which have been pushed down into the Id by repression, are virtually immortal and are preserved for whole decades as though they had only recently occurred (Freud, 1949).

But, they can be made conscious in analytic treatment.

Morality is unknown to the Id and in general the Id knows no values. The instinctual impulses of the Id are plentifully provided with energy; they are plastic and capable of attaching themselves to objects in several ways. Consider dreams and the numerous ways Id impulses find expression through them. Freud wrote that the quantitative, energic factor, closely allied to the Pleasure Principle, dominates all the processes of the Id. (So, it would appear, that he was unable to formulate in any intelligible fashion how destructive drives operate there).

The blind impulsions of the Id striving for gratification would cause the self-destruction of the individual — if he could survive infancy — were it not for the fact that the Ego has taken over the task of representing the external world to the Id. Since the Ego is the seat of intelligence, it has the task of modifying — but never abandoning — the Pleasure Principle. The Ego controls the paths to action on behalf of the Id, while it interpolates thought between desire and action, making possible reflection, with the help of past experience. "In popular language," Freud wrote, "we may say that the Ego stands for reason and circumspection, while the Id stands for the untamed passions (Freud, 1949).

PSYCHOSEXUAL DEVELOPMENT

Freud taught that sexuality does not first appear at puberty, but at the beginning of life, developing through manifold stages: oral; anal (or anal-sadistic); phallic, with a hiatus called the latency period; and puberty, which introduces and merges with adolescence. In order to make this "theory" intelligible, Freud postulated the existence of a qualitatively special kind of energy at the disposal of the instincts, called libido. It is important to realize that the pleasure derived from the operation of this energy at any stage has an erotic quality, not to be confused with any and every pleasure in the popular sense. The libido exists in every part of the body. Hence, stimulation of any part of the body is capable of arousing erotic pleasure.

It is important to mention that there were numerous and rich sources for Freud's conceptions of sexuality to be found in the literature of his day and, frequently, in the practices of people living in Continental Europe. These matters are described in Ellenberger's great scholarly work *The Discovery of the Unconscious* (Ellenberger, 1970). Therefore, it is not surprising that in searching for a psychological model of the neuroses, Freud borrowed heavily from the literary and cultural climate of his day. Equally important, perhaps, was the fact that Freud's female patients, who suffered from hysterical neuroses, were richly endowed with intense sexual repressions which seemed to produce a bewildering array of symptoms. In describing such symptoms, Freud's great contemporary from whom he seems to have borrowed a good deal, Pierre Janet, could exercise his considerable literary gifts, as did Freud. But it is worth noting that Janet rejected Freud's psychological model (Ellenberger, 1970).

Oral Stage

In the course of the oral stage, the infant derives erotic pleasure from eating, sucking, and activities connected with the mouth in general. Freud also claimed that a child's first erotic object is the mother's breast. The child cannot perceive himself separated from the mother's breast and hence in the words of Margaret Mahler (1952) forms a "kind of social symbiosis."

Anal Stage

During the anal phase, which begins roughly around the age of one and a half years, the infant (child, if one prefers) derives erotic pleasure first from the elimination of the contents of the bladder and bowel, and, in the second phase, from withholding them. Freud does not seem to have fully

The phylogenetic foundation has so much the upper hand in all this over accidental experience that it makes no difference whether a child has really sucked at the breast or has been brought up on the bottle and never enjoyed the tenderness of a mother's care. His development takes the same path in both cases; it may be that in the latter event his later longing is all the greater (Freud, 1949).

Sullivan's theories on these matters will be compared and discussed later.

Freud has also speculated that the castration dread which often terrifies little boys also has a phylogenetic memory-trace going back to certain events of a Primal Horde existing long before the dawn of history. These matters are clarified in his book *Totem and Taboo*. The Oedipus Complex is a part of man's constitution. Ultimately, failure to resolve the Oedipus Complex, the kernel of every neurosis, reflected the inborn strength of the libidinal drive that was directed at the mother. This failure was due to a phylogenetic inheritance as noted above, going back to the events of an original Primal Horde (as described in *Totem and Taboo*), the source of a primal Oedipus Complex. The basic idea in this book is that long before the dawn of history there existed a Primal Horde ruled by an all-powerful father who kept all the women to himself. At some point in this prehistoric period, the sons rebelled, slew and ate the father in order to keep the mother and daughters for themselves. But, in order to avoid chaotic conflict, they created a barrier against possession of their mothers and sisters, which became the Superego. Leaving aside many important details, one must be aware that the Oedipus Complex and the associated guilt for this crime was supposedly recapitulated in every succeeding generation.

During the phallic phase, the sexuality of boys and girls divides. The threat of the castration dread forces the boy to repress and, in the most normal cases, resolve the Oedipus Complex, while the Superego takes its place. This occurs as the boy identifies with his father and, as previously mentioned, adopts or introjects his father's ideals. It may happen that a residue of the boy's erotic fixation to his mother will remain in the form of an extensive dependence on her, continuing through life as an attitude of subjection toward women. The effects of the castration dread are said to be many and incalculable, affecting the whole of the boy's relations with his parents and, subsequently, with men and women in general. How much damage is done by the threat of castration and how much is avoided seems to depend on "quantitative" relations. If a strong feminine component exists in the boy, the threat to his masculinity is increased, and he falls into a passive attitude toward his father such as he ascribes to his mother. In fact, Freud ascribed a psychological bisexuality to everyone, although normally either masculine or feminine components are uppermost.

been aware that this second phase of the anal stage may be related to the child's efforts at gaining attention and love. Another development during this stage is an intense aggressive drive, although the oral stage has an aggressive component as well.

Phallic Stage (Oedipus Complex of the Boy)

The third stage of development is called the phallic stage, which in boys is contemporaneous with the Oedipus Complex. At about the age of two and a half or three years every little boy begins to form a sexual attachment to his mother. He likes to kiss her, caress her, watch her undress, and sleep with her at night. At the same time, he begins to regard his father, whom he has been previously fond of, as a rival whom he would like to get rid of. But, he cannot enjoy this romance for long, although he may substitute an older sister for his mother. Unless he has a constitutional predisposition towards a fixation at this stage (or a very distrubed mother who may sleep in the same bed with her son every night, as in one of Sullivan's "cases," until about age 21, when he had to be placed in a mental hospital), he must resolve (roughly repress) his sexual attachment to his mother, chiefly owing to the castration dread (a fear of having the penis cut off). He then progresses into a period or phase of latency where the development of the libidinal drive slows down or ceases temporarily. On successful resolution of the Oedipus Complex, the boy sublimates his attachment to his mother and feels tenderly toward her.

Up until the pubertal phase, the sexual drive is composed of several "streams," components which then unite to form one main stream or drive under the primacy of the genital zone. Normally, the incestuous wishes remain repressed, if they have not been abandoned, and the individual seeks out a "foreign object," a non-incestual object of the opposite sex whom the boy can "love" in reality.

The intensity of the Oedipus Complex is prefigured by the fact that a child's first erotic object is the mother's breast that feeds him. In its beginnings, love (erotic pleasure) is said to attach itself to the satisfaction of the need for food. In the beginning, the infant does not perceive the breast as separate from him. The mother's (or her surrogate's) breast subsequently becomes fused or completed into the whole person of the mother, who feeds him, takes care of him, and thus, arouses in him many other pleasant and unpleasant sensations. This leads to some basic divergencies between Freud and Sullivan. Freud wrote:

> By her care of the child's body she becomes his first seducer. In these two relations lies the root of a mother's importance, unique, without parallel, laid down unalterably for a whole lifetime, as the first and strongest love-object and as the prototype of all later love relations — for both sexes.

FEMININE PSYCHOLOGY

Feminine psychology has not fared well in classical psychoanalysis. One gets the impression that Freud regarded women as the inferior sex — despite his protestations that this was not so.

Freud looked upon the psychology of women as a "riddle." He asserted that both sexes seem to pass through the early phases of sexual development in the same way. During the anal-sadistic phase, little girls are as aggressive as little boys. In the anal-sadistic phase, the little girls, like the little boy, is "a little man." Like the little boy, she discovers how to obtain pleasurable sensations from manipulation of her even smaller clitoris which is supposedly a penis equivalent. If this notion seems strange to the reader, one must realize that Freud believed that there is only one sexual organ for the child, the penis; the clitoris at this time is a penis equivalent. The little girl's first love object is also her mother. However, in the Oedipus situation, she regards her father as her love object. Now she has to change her erotogenic zone (clitoris to vagina) and her object (from mother to father).

How then does the little girl pass from her masculine phase, characterized by intense aggressive as well as passive wishes, to the feminine, which is chiefly characterized by passive aims? In short, until she enters the Oedipus situation, her libidinal relations to her mother pass through all the phases of infantile sexuality, taking on the attributes of each phase. Thus, for Freud, femininity goes through a circuitous development, based upon the model of the male. There is only one sexual organ, the penis, for the clitoris is a stunted penis. In *New Introductory Lectures on Psychoanalysis*, Freud (1949) wrote:

> There is only one libido which is as much in the service of the male as of the female sexual function. ...the phrase "feminine libido" cannot possibly be justified.

Oedipus Complex of the Girl

If the preceding is so, why is it that the girl turns away from her mother, frequently in an atmosphere of hate, to her father? In her case, the castration dread is crucially important, although, in a sense, different from that of the boy.

> The castration-complex in the girl, as well, is started by the sight of the genital organs of the other sex. She immediately notices the difference, and. . .its significance. She feels herself at a great disadvantage, and often declares that she would "like to have something like that too" and falls a victim to penis-envy, which leaves ineradicable traces on her development and character-formation, and even in the most favorable instances, is not overcome without a great deal of expenditure of mental energy (Freud, 1949).

Years later, as psychoanalysis has allegedly proved, Freud wrote, this desire for a penis will persist in her unconscious, retaining a considerable amount of energy. Thus, the desires of women to pursue intellectual interests such as becoming a psychoanalyst, a physician, a lawyer, or an engineer, can often be recognized as a sublimated modification of this repressed wish.

The discovery of her castration is said to be a turning point in the life of the girl. Her discovery of her castration causes her enjoyment of phallic sexuality, to be spoiled by the influence of penis envy. Freud asserts that she is wounded in her self-love by the unfavorable comparison with the boy "who is so much better equipped," and therefore, normally gives up the masturbatory satisfaction which she obtained from her clitoris, while she repudiates her love for her mother and at the same time, often represses a good deal of her sexual impulses in general. The little girl's passive side now gains the upper hand. At the same time, she turns to her father from whom she now wishes to obtain a penis, "which her mother has refused her." The feminine situation is said to be established only when the wish for the penis is replaced by the wish for a child in accordance with the old pre-Oedipal wish, to impregnate the mother with child, as well as the corresponding one to have a child by the mother. As in the case of the little boy, her mother is her first seducer.

The girl enters into the situation of the Oedipus Complex with the transference of the child-penis wish to her father. Since her fear of castration has disappeared, the most powerful motive for the resolution of the Oedipus Complex does not exist. Freud asserts that the girl remains in the Oedipus situation for an indefinite period, abandoning it late in life and then incompletely. Her father is her first choice; her husband is at best a second. Freud believed that this desire for a child by the father results in great happiness in later life if she bears a child by her husband or lover, especially if the child is a little boy who brings the longed-for penis with him.

According to Freud, the Superego of women is feeble. In men, powerful factors exist which will normally, in the course of experience, make possible the development of a more or less rigorous conscience. This has already been dealt with at length in previous portions of this chapter. Education and threats of loss of love must suffice in the development of a woman's conscience. When the Oedipus Complex passes away, the child (the boy, at any rate) must abandon the intense attachments to his parents. In the case of the boy, identification seems to compensate for the loss of his sexual attachment to his mother. Identifications with the parents or at least one of them becomes greatly intensified—at least for the boy. But, for reasons already mentioned, the more feeble Superego of the girl cannot attain the strength and independence which gives it its cultural significance.

Bisexuality and Femininity

It has been briefly mentioned previously that Freud adopted the notion of bisexuality. This had been suggested to him by a friend. According to Freud, from a biological point of view, both sexes share similar attributes to a considerable degree. In particular, parts of the male sexual apparatus are also to be found in the body of the female, although in a rudimentary condition, and vice versa. Freud professed to be puzzled as to how one might characterize femininity and masculinity psychologically. But, despite many disclaimers and qualifications, he tended to attribute active aims to men and more or less passive aims to women. Yet, he reminds us (as female analysts reminded him) that social conventions also force women into passive substitutions. Hence, both their constitutions, childhood experiences, and social norms impose repression of women's aggressiveness, and the development of strong masochistic impulses as well. (Masochism is basically the sexual enjoyment of psychic pain inflicted by the partner. Sadism is fundamentally the sexual enjoyment of inflicting psychic pain.)

> Masochism is then. . .truly feminine. But when, as so often happens, you meet with masochism in men, what else can you do but say that these men display obvious feminine traits of character (Freud, 1949).

By and large, normal women tend to be more or less passive and masochistic, while men tend to be aggressive and perhaps sadistic.

SULLIVAN'S ADAPTATIONAL ORIENTATION

In their masterly paper *A Methodological Study of Freudian Theory*, Kardiner, Karush and Ovesey (1966) performed a precise, logical, and historical analysis of Freudian psychology. They distinguish between the Freudian instinctual framework and their own "adaptational frame of reference."

By and large, Sullivan's psychology may be called adaptational, a frame of reference which goes back at least to William James. Sullivan completely abandoned the so-called libido theory, although for a brief period, he equated it with "hormic energy" perhaps because he was moderately influenced by the hormic psychology of William McDougall, a very able contributor to the field of psychology during the early part of this century. For Sullivan, the energy he talked about during most of his career is the energy of physics which can assume various forms. He abandoned Freud's formulation of psychosexual development, although he retained several features of it, stripped of their libidinal underpinnings. While he learned a great deal from Freud's psychoanalytic techniques, he reinterpreted them, modified them, and created techniques of his own as his work with patients dictated. In contrast to the founder of psychoanalysis, who began his psychoanalytic career working with female neurotic patients, Sullivan dealt mainly with schizophrenic patients during the early part of his career, particularly schizophrenic youths and young men. Unfortunately, Sullivan died when he was fifty-seven, apparently at the peak of his career.

Sullivan wrote only one book, *Personal Psychopathology*, which he finished somewhere around 1932—but he never published it. Why, is not certainly clear. However, it was published in mimeograph form in 1965 and in book form in 1972. The other books of Sullivan contain various lecture series he delivered over the years and have been comprehensively edited.

Basic Conceptions

The subject of Sullivanian psychology is human performances, including revery processes and thought, which can be characterized by their end-states or goals. These performances can be categorized into a two-part classification, the pursuit of satisfactions or, in other words, the satisfaction of physiological drives, and the pursuit of security. The first classification will be familiar to the reader; the second may not be quite as clear. Thus, the pursuit of satisfactions pertains to the fulfillment of needs which are rather closely connected with the bodily organization of man.

The pursuit of security, Sullivan said, pertains rather more closely to man's cultural equipment than to his somatic organization. Needless to say, the "cultural equipment" of man throughout the world is what the anthropologist studies; it is his peculiar field, rather than a study of the fine arts. In 1940 when Sullivan "published" his first series of lectures that later became the book, *Conceptions of Modern Psychiatry*, in the journal, "Psychiatry," virtually nothing was known about heredity, or at least very little. No matter how important this topic may be, not much will be said about it in this book. Apart from his limitations of knowledge, Sullivan's interests were mainly concerned with a different area of human life. But, it is quite clear that Sullivan would regard a knowledge of biochemistry, or of the endocrine glands, or the nervous system as no more than tributary to an understanding of functional mental disorders, or, as he subsequently called them, difficulties in living. (In this connection, it should be noted that Sullivan regarded the differences between mental disorder and mental health as only one of degree). That is what psychopathology is all about, difficulties in living—even the organic psychoses.

Why Sullivan employed "security" to label the field which is almost synonymous with social psychology will presently become clear. As for individual psychology, to which Gordon Allport and others have devoted so much time and energy, Sullivan taught that it is beyond the reach of scientific study—although in actual fact he could not strictly adhere to this point of view. *Individuality* has several meanings—and that can be confusing if one is not clear about it. But *human* individuality has a special meaning of its own, quite different from any other (See Sullivan, 1950).

As for the meaning of *security*, Sullivan asserted in a lecture he gave around 1939:

> This second class, the pursuit of security, may be regarded as consisting of ubiquitous artifacts—again in the anthropological sense, manmade— evolved by the cultural conditioning or training; that is, education of the impulses or drives which underlie the first class. In other words, given our biological equipment—we are bound to need food and water and so on—certain conditioning influences can be brought to bear on the needs for satisfaction. And the cultural conditioning gives rise to the second group, the second great class of interpersonal phenomena, the pursuit of security (Sullivan, 1953).

In this lecture, Sullivan also introduced a fundamental concept of contemporary psychiatry which stirred up a great deal of controversy. The infant's striving for ability, for power and competence as Sullivan said:

> The full development of personality along the lines of security is chiefly founded on infant's discovery of his powerlessness to achieve certain desired end states. . .From the disappointments in the very early stages of life outside the womb. . . . comes the beginning of this vast development of actions, thoughts, foresights and so on (Sullivan, 1953).

This concept may have been one of the basic cornerstones for Melanie Klein's orientation and later the contemporary ego psychology. The notion that every human being has a built-in striving for power— however innocently meant—was obnoxious to psychoanalysts of European origin. The term "power" lent itself too easily to misinterpretation. In subsequent years, Sullivan virtually ignored this formulation, since he lived long enough to redefine it.

Man is born virtually helpless, and for many years cannot survive without the care and nurture of his parents or their surrogates, with whose help he learns a vast number of things even before he starts formal education. The developing actions, thoughts, foresights, and so on

> are calculated to protect one from feelings of insecurity and helplessness in the situation which confronts one. This accultural evolution begins thus, and when it succeeds, when one evolves successfully along this line, then one respects oneself, and as one respects oneself so one can respect others (Sullivan, 1953).

"As you judge yourself, so shall you judge others," (Sullivan, 1953), consciously or otherwise, and not conversely. For Sullivan, this is a fundamental assumption of human personality. Self-respect, a conviction that one has the attributes which merit the approval of others owing to one's past experience, and one's achievements, contributes substantially toward self-confidence and the ability to do the things which evoke the esteem of others, as well as a legitimate, realistic pride in oneself.

But, self-respect, and the competence which flows from it, do not grow overnight. It is the acculturation or education by the parents, especially the one who mothers, which at first fosters self-respect or self-esteem in the offspring. The feelings, attitudes, and actions of the mothering one as she fulfills her role as the one who mothers and fulfills the infant's needs, especially during the early years of life, are most vital in the development of a healthy, self-assured person. Subsequent experiences in school are also of great importance but, to a great extent, they foster or inhibit, or even destroy the budding personality, that is the "marvelous characteristics" of a normal, healthy child. These matters will be explicated in detail throughout later chapters.

REFERENCES

Ariette, S. (ed). *The American Handbook of Psychiatry.* Vol. 1, pp. 816–840 Basic Books, New York, 1959.

Cooley, C. *Social Organization.* Scribner and Sons, New York, 1909.

Cooley, C. *Human Nature and the Social Order.* Scribner and Sons, New York, 1922.

Edel, A. *The Theory and Practice of Philosophy, Part III: What Is A Man?* Harcourt, Brace, and Jovanovich, New York, 1946.

Ellenberger, H.F. *The Discovery of the Unconscious.* Basic Books, New York, 1970.

Freud, S. *A General Introduction to Psychoanalysis.* Garden City Publishing, New York, 1943.

Freud, S. *New Introductory Lectures on Psychoanalysis.* W.W. Norton, New York, 1949.

Freud, S. *An Outline of Psychoanalysis,* trans. by James Strachey. W.W. Norton, New York, 1949.

Green, A. *Sociology.* McGraw-Hill, New York, 1952.

Havens, L.L. *Approaches to the Mind.* Little, Brown and Company, Boston, 1973.

James, W. *The Principles of Psychology.* 2 Vols. Henry Holt, New York, 1907.

Kardiner, A., Karush, A., and Ovesey, L. A methodological study of Freudian theory. *Int. J. Psychiatr.* 1966; 2: 489.

Klein, M. *Comprehensive Textbook of Psychiatry,* Third Ed., Vol. 1. Williams and Wilkins, Baltimore, 1980.

Luce, G.G., and Segal, J. *Sleep.* Coward–McCann, New York, 1949.

Mahler, M. On child psychosis and schizophrenia, in *The Psychoanalytic Study of the Child.* International Univ. Press, New York, 1952.

Mullahy, P. *Psychoanalysis and Interpersonal Psychiatry.* Science House, New York, 1970.

Ruch, F., and Zimbardo, P.G. *Psychology and Life,* 8th Ed., Scott, Foresman and Company, Glenview, Ill., 1971.

Salzman, L. *Developments in Psychoanalysis*. Grune and Stratton, New York, 1962.
Sartain, A., North, A., Strange, J., and Chapman, H. *Psychology: Understanding Human Behavior*. McGraw-Hill, New York, 1973.
Schachtel, E. *Metamorphosis*. Basic Books, New York, 1959.
Sullivan, H.S. The illusion of personal individuality. *Psychiatry*. 1950; 13: 317–332.
Sullivan, H.S. *Conceptions of Modern Psychiatry*. W.W. Norton, New York, 1953.
Sullivan, H.S. *Personal Psychopathology*. W.W. Norton, New York, 1972.

2

The Totality of
Organism and Environment

THE CELL (TRANSACTIONISM)

As Sullivan clearly stated in *Conceptions of Modern Psychiatry* (1953), it is artificial to say that the living cell in the uterus is one thing, and its necessary environment another. He asserted that the cell manifests the basic categories of biological process. Its potentialities are almost "stupefying." Although the cell is a demonstrable entity, it lives and starts the realization of its potentialities living "communally" with, or by means of, the uterine environment. This environment, from a relative position in time and space, flows through the living cell, becoming of its very life in the process. And the cell "flows and grows through the environment, establishing in this process its particular career-line as an organism". Since Sullivan put great emphasis on the organization of personality, it seems wise to stress the importance of organization at every phase of the organism's growth. He stated:

> Before there are any elaborate differentiations of tissue, however, before in fact there has been a single division of the fertile cell, there is organization in the cell-medium complex, such that a vital balance is maintained in the more purely organismic part of the complex (Sullivan, 1953).

Summarily, Sullivan thought that, biologically, an organism is a self-perpetuating organization of the physico-chemical world which manifests life by functional activity in the complex.

Heredity and Maturation

In roughly one generation since Sullivan delivered the lectures in "Psychiatry" published as *Conceptions of Modern Psychiatry* in 1953, biology and its sub-branches have made extraordinary strides. In the

1930's, as already stated, there was relatively little knowledge of the internal environment of the cell.

Before proceeding further, however, it is important to mention the elementary distinction between heredity and maturation. *Heredity* is "the direction and pattern given by the genes to growth and development." *Maturation* is "the completion of growth and development within the organism." (Sartain et al., 1973) It is also important to remember the importance of the *physical environment* of the organism during the course of its growth. Sartain et al. (1973) point out that every organ and system within the body must mature over a period of time before it is ready to function. Although most organs are able to function at birth, some of the organs and systems are farther along the path of development than others.

In addition to heredity and maturation, factor of time, biologically and psychologically, must not be ignored. Sartain et al. (1973) provide us with a good perspective from which to start. (Subsequently, the importance of time in the organism's development as a person will have to be emphasized.)

> In the process of maturation, we see the interaction of heredity and environment over the course of time. For example, a girl's ovaries are not mature enough to produce fully ripened eggs until she reaches puberty, which comes ordinarily between the years of eleven and fifteen. However, a number of environmental changes and conditions can affect the onset of puberty. Malnutrition, chronic illness and serious emotional instability can all slow this maturation process. A girl in a war-torn country without sufficient food may not reach puberty until she is twenty years old (Sartain et al., 1973).

It is a well-known fact in medicine that girls in different countries, climates, and cultures reach puberty at different ages.

THE FOUR GENERIC FACTORS

Sullivan stated that there are four different generic factors which enter into any person's actions: biological potentiality, its level of maturation, the "results" obtained by previous experience, and "foresight" or anticipation of the future. In regard to the first two, their meaning is reasonably clear. The third generic factor's related primarily to the period which extends shortly after birth to any given moment in a person's life. The clinician has to learn a great deal about what happened to his client or "patient," for example, in the course of his investigation as to "what ails the patient." Past experience is cumulative, and makes us what we are now, given a biological substrate. Most of this book will directly, or indirectly, deal with this matter.

Foresight is not limited to sporadic incidents of our lives. It is a constant companion, usually semi-unconscious. At any given moment, we stand, Janus-like, facing the past and the prospective future—although we are not ordinarily conscious of this fact.

In the discussion of human potentialities and their development in a suitable, or at least more or less adequate environment, through time, nothing directly was said about biological and human needs. To be sure, the outline of Freudian psychology dealt extensively with certain inherently biological needs as they became manifest stage by stage. For the sake of clarity, it is necessary to stress the difference between somatic ("biological") and cultural needs. But, in actual fact, they interlock; they become interrelated. So much so, that the human (cultural) needs which are acquired for the most part during the fairly long stretch of time from infancy to adulthood "invade" the somatic apparatus during the *process of acculturation*. It is a commonplace that the human infant at birth is relatively helpless. Sullivan used to say that the young infant's mightiest tool is the cry which introduces subsequent learning. Since we apparently have no instincts—in the strict sense—we have to learn how to live and how to be or become a fully human being.

It should be emphasized that Sullivan did not attempt to superimpose man's socio-cultural development on a fixed biological or psychosexual framework in the manner of Erik Erikson in *Childhood and Society* (Erikson, 1950). Just as it is "artificial" to separate the organism from its physico-chemical environment, it is equally superficial to separate the individual from his socio-cultural environment.

EUPHORIA AND TENSION

Absolute euphoria is a state of utter, tensionless well-being, which never exists in reality. The human organism is constantly bombarded with stimuli from the outside world and from within. The central nervous system is always in some state of tension, which is needed for the screening of these stimuli. One is only tensionless when he is dead. Hence, absolute euphoria is a construct design to organize thought.

Sullivan suggested that the nearest approach to anything like what one may observe is possibly that of a very young infant in a state of deep sleep. Of course, he did not imply that normal, healthy people yearn for infantile bliss. It is biologically essential to maintain an indefinitely specifiable rhythmic level of tension, analogous to the Pleasure Principle of Freud but by no means identical with, primarily because pleasure is *not* what people ordinarily strive for. The Freudian Pleasure Principle comes under the label of psychological hedonism. Of the many difficulties raised by the latter, Gordon Allport has pointed out that one cannot aim directly at the achievement of pleasure or happiness.

> Someone may *think* that if he obtains a college degree, marries Susan, earns a good living, he will be happy; but these *concrete* accomplishments are the tangible goals. Happiness is at best a by-product of otherwise motivated activity. One who aims at happiness has no aim at all (Allport, 1961).

Sullivan asserted that absolute tension might be defined as the maximum possible deviation from *absolute euphoria*. He also said that the nearest approach to absolute tension that one observes is the rather uncommon, and always relatively transient, state of terror. Hence, absolute tension is also a construct, merely related to absolute euphoria.

Tension of Somatic Needs

Sullivan held that those tensions that episodically or recurrently lower the level of the infant's euphoria (or well-being) and effect the "biologic disequilibration" of his being are needs—needs pertaining to his "communal existence" with the physico-chemical world. It is the communal existence of the organism which brings about the imbalance. Just as one needs the solid ground to walk upon, one needs oxygen to breathe, food to eat, water to drink, etc. Hence, as previously noted, we live by means of the envirnoment. Apart from this transaction, it is not possible to understand human existence.

Tension of Cultural Needs

Since man is a bio-socio-cultural being, the definition of all somatic needs has to be supplemented. The environment is socio-cultural as well as physical. Both make up a transaction. It is in relation to the framework of man's socio-cultural environment that human relations, interpersonal relations, occur as they are structured by the family, school, and other socio-cultural institutions. Hence, the socio-cultural dimension introduces another class of needs, which Sullivan characterized variously as his career progressed—needs for self-esteem or self-respect, or in other words, needs for interpersonal security. Failure to fulfil one or more of either of the two classes of needs causes a lowering of euphoria, an increase in tension. What was called cultural needs are often called acquired or learned needs. However, due to genetic and environmental factors, individual variations among human beings are incalculably numerous. But, in any given community or society, the sociocultural framework sets limits beyond which individuals who attempt to surmount them have often encountered lethal hostility, at least in a stable society. The twentieth century has provided us with numerous examples of what may happen when a society, owing to wars, and revolutions and counterrevolutions following upon wars, suffers the destruction of its traditions.

The Tension of Sleep

In addition, the tensions of somatic needs and of anxiety (or of the needs for interpersonal security) are "oppositional" to the needs for sleep. We know that one of the major vegetative (somatic) signs of severe depression and anxiety states is insomnia. Early in the schizophrenic decompansation, the patient will complain of severe insomnia. The student who is anxious because of an examination may sleep poorly because of the individual meaning of that examination usually in the sphere of interpersonal security.

THE DEVELOPMENTAL ERAS

Sullivan constructed a much more elaborate formulation of human development than did Freud. He chose the same starting point as did the latter, namely the *oral zone*. In *The Interpersonal Theory of Psychiatry* (Sullivan, 1953) Sullivan subjected this zone to a much more thorough analysis than did Freud himself, which includes a brief discussion of the neurophysiological substrate involved in the act of sucking. Normally, the infant gains satisfaction when his need for food is fulfilled by the act of sucking either at the mother's breast or from the nipple of a bottle containing the appropriate formula. Borrowing a suggestion from the psychiatrist David Levy, Sullivan postulated the existence, as a rule, of an excess of energy to perform the act of sucking. In other words, nature generally provides the infant with more than sufficient energy for this task, which is necessary to survival. In order to get rid of the excess energy, the baby will suck his thumb or almost anything available within reach. Pleasure may be a result of this activity, but it seems to have nothing to do with an hypothetical libidinal energy.

One of the special reflexes the child is born with is the sucking reflex. Touching a finger to the infants mouth elicits this reflex. This reflex diminishes after a few months and is absent after one year. The infant's mouth is built and equipped in a way that enables him to continue his attachment to a feeding source after the umbilical cord is cut. Sucking, apart from satisfying the appetite of the infant, has a major role in helping the child to recognize deprivation and gratification. Sucking has a reality function linking the infant more and more to the outer world. It is not surprising, that this inner space of primary importance is equipped with the most sophisticated and mature organ at birth. The tongue is endowed with multiple senses—temperature, pain, touch, deep sensations, and taste, and asserts voluntary and involuntary control over those who would relate to the mouth. Survival of a species depends on careful guarding of the inner space, so judgement and instinct of the maturing infant determine when the muscles guarding that space relax to permit entrance.

Sullivan wrote that from the beginning of the breathing cycle the infant has a "whole list" of needs, activities and satisfactions. Delays in satisfactions, he added, constitute dangers to early infantile survival, which become a source of augmented tension which he called a fear-like state, one that he carefully distinguished from anxiety tension as the infant matures. Normally, or very frequently, crying is an adequate and appropriate action to bring about the relief of fear because crying causes the mothering one to "rally round" and engage in the necessary form of tender behavior which removes the source of tension. Very early in life—exactly how early is not known at this stage in child psychology —the infant's experiences of crying-when-hungry, or crying-when-thirsty or crying-in-pain, etc., and the ensuing relief, become the basis of at least elementary recall and foresight. The infant, in a rudimentary fashion, at first, learns to relate backward and forward.

Infrequently the crying-when-hungry, for example, does not bring relief because at the moment there is no one present ot act tenderly or take care of the particular need appropriately. When this happens in normal, healthy homes, the infant may fall asleep for a while and the hunger is alleviated temporarily and then he may wake up crying again. When the tension of needs is markedly aggravated, whether it be due to hunger, thirst, or fear, the infant lapses into apathy, wherein all the tensions of *needs* are markedly attenuated. This implies that the infant's vital processes are slowed down so that if he is in some dire situation in which apathy is prolonged he may die. Direct observations of infants deprived of the attention of a suitable mothering figure reveal a syndrome that is termed in contemporary literature as Anaclitic Depression. In this syndrome, the infant goes through a characteristic sequence of changes including protest (intense crying and struggling) which leads to a phase of despair. Some of these infants fail to thrive, may stop eating and waste away and die (1953). When they survive, they become detached, withdrawn from human relations, and preoccupied with inanimate objects, body parts, masturbation, fecal smearing, "head banging," and rocking (Lynn 1980). The syndrome of Anaclitic

Depression has been foreshadowed by Sullivan's "apathy," which was described by him as a detached "sleep-like state" that results from neglect and the induction of fear due to lack of the "mothering one."

Although Sullivan was not too sure about it, he thought it likely that another syndrome in infancy, a protective dynamism called somnolent detachment, may appear. Somnolent detachment is described in Sullivan's *Interpersonal Theory of Psychiatry* (1953).

THE POSTULATE OF TENDERNESS

The care of the young can never be accomplished in an impersonal fashion. As Sullivan has said, it is not a matter of procuring a bigger and better incubator; nor are the biological changes that occur during pregnancy, delivery, and post partum sufficient to explain mothering behavior. In human beings, the "biology" of the mother is by no means sufficient to account for tender behavior, expecially when it extends over a period of many years. This is poignantly clear when one realizes that the biological father may be the parent who does the mothering. The "mothering one" may be a relative, or an individual who has no blood relationship to the infant. It is well established that a great deal of learning (of experience which fosters tenderness) has to be acquired, even in the case of the mother. In human males, there appear to be no innately occurring hormones or other biochemical factors which would foster mothering behavior, although this is not definitely established in some animal species. Moreover, current research shows that in some strains of rats one can prevent females from retrieving pups by testosterone treatment (Quadagno et al., 1973). As far as is known, the human paternal drive is a result of learning, which is mainly cultural (Ciba, 1975), or what Skinner would call conditioning.

On the basis of his postulates on parental behavior, Sullivan formulated a principle or theorem which runs as follows:

> The observed activity of the infant arising from the tension of needs induces tension in the mothering one, which tension is experienced as tenderness and as an impulsion to activities toward the relief of the infant's needs (Sullivan, 1953).

The baby's crying-when-hungry, for example, elicits tender behavior by the mothering one. This is what normally or very frequently occurs. And so it is with the care of the infant's various other needs the mothering one "rallies round" and acts to relieve the infant's distress.

From the recurrent experiences of tenderness, the infant gradually develops a class of tensions which may be labeled "need for tenderness."

The class of needs to act tenderly is complementary to the class of tensions called "need for tenderness." Moreover, the infant's recurrent experience of tenderness will eventually create another class of tensions in him: *The need to act tenderly*. Children's playing with dolls seems to provide a clue to their incipient education in how to act tenderly. Depending on a variety of circumstances, including the steadfast tenderness of parents toward the offspring, the generic need to act tenderly is fostered or thwarted over a period of a good many years.

Contemporary research of mother-infant relationships supports these original ideas of Sullivan. Mother-infant relationship consists of transaction sequences of both infant and mothering one affecting each other, and research in this field should address itself to both (Ciba, 1975).

There is no necessary connection between "romantic love," which is essentially sublimated sexually, and tenderness. Since the latter is closely linked up with the family, whether nuclear, extended, etc., it is clearly related not only to the structure and quality of family life, but to social institutions generally. This is one reason that Sullivanian theory always tempts one to trespass on the domains of sociology, anthropology, and ancillary fields of study. For such a reason, among others, Sullivan advocated an interdisciplinary approach.

FREUD'S CONCEPTIONS OF ANXIETY

Freud's formulations of anxiety can be roughly distinguished into *two stages*. In his earlier writings, he thought that the birth trauma constitutes the prototype for the state of anxiety. The process of birth evokes in mental experience a condition of intense excitation or tension which is felt as pain. Regardless of the validity of this idea, it is important to remember that anxiety always is correlated with tension. Since Freud attempted to formulate anxiety-tension within the framework of the Pleasure Principle, he encountered many difficulties.

Freud's second formulation of anxiety is linked up with the division of the personality into Id, Ego, and Superego. The ego "is the only seat of anxiety." It alone can produce and feel anxiety. But what is the anxiety all about? Danger. Danger from where and from what? Before attempting to answer such a question, it is important to mention that there is still a suggestion of the original formulation of the source of the anxiety state. The birth of a baby has its dangers. Be that as it may, before the latest formulation of the tripartite division of the mind, Freud had distinguished three main varieties of anxiety: objective anxiety, neurotic anxiety, and moral anxiety. The new formulation of personality structure enabled Freud to relate the dependence of the Ego on the external world, the Id and the Superego. Anxiety and fear are so closely related in Freud's theory that one cannot clearly distinguish them. Anxiety had long been thought of as a signal indicating the presence of danger. In other words, the feeling of fear serves as a warning that danger, whether from without or within, is present. Brenner (1955) has lucidly summed up the meaning of this statement: In the course of growth,

> "the young child learns to anticipate the advent of a traumatic situation and to react to it with anxiety before it becomes traumatic (painful or injurious). This type of anxiety Freud called "signal anxiety." It is produced by a situation of *danger* or the anticipation of danger, its production is a function of the ego, and it serves to mobilize the forces at the command of the ego to meet or to avoid the impending traumatic situation."

Since the Ego's chief function is self preservation, external danger arouses fear (or anxiety), a condition in which there is considerable tension or excitation. According to Freud, this "reality anxiety" merges imperceptibly with "neurotic anxiety," a fear of instinctual demands or Id impulses, from which one cannot flee. Freud believed that failure to resolve the Oedipus Complex, which for him is biological and universally ordained, is the kernel of every neurosis. He also wrote that neurotic people remain infantile in their attitudes toward danger. They never outgrow infantile fears, such as castration dread or the fear of loss of love and object (person) loss. Moral anxiety is said to be a fear of the harsh Superego, which can punish one with painful feelings of guilt.

Neurotic anxiety and moral anxiety are related to reality anxiety. Freud wrote that normally the fear of the Superego should never cease, since it is indispensable in social relations in the form of moral anxiety. This fear is based on a realistic factor. The violation of the moral code of a community has always been fraught with danger. Neurotic anxiety is the fear that the instincts will prove too powerful, too intense and demanding, and get out of control (by failure of defensive operations for example), causing the individual to perform acts for which he will be punished. This too has a basis in reality. Every society has set certain limits to the gratification of instinctual drives. If one oversteps those limits one exposes oneself to danger. However, neurotic persons have childish fears and magnify and distort possible dangers. They also imagine dangers and punishments which do not exist. Reality danger is self-explanatory, although the individual has to learn what the realistic dangers of the world are and how to cope.

There is one final point to be raised about Freud's formulations of anxiety. If the Ego employs anxiety as a signal of danger, and if, at the same time, anxiety is a signal to the Ego that a danger situation exists, is not this self-contradictory? Whether Freud himself saw this problem is uncertain. But Brenner is very clear about it and tries to resolve it. He asserts that the Ego is a *group of related functions*. "We believe," he wrote,

> that in a danger situation certain of these functions, e.g., sensory perception, memory, and some type of thought process, are concerned with recognizing the danger, while other parts of the Ego; or other Ego functions react to the danger with what is perceived as anxiety (Brenner, 1955).

In this statement, it seems, Brenner has extricated Freud from several pseudo problems.

SULLIVAN'S CONCEPTIONS OF ANXIETY

Sullivan seems to have attributed more importance to anxiety than even Freud. Although Sullivan is indebted to Freud, he interpreted anxiety within a different framework. Just as we have omitted several details of Freud's formulations, we will omit several details about the same topic which are discussed in Sullivan's *Conceptions of Modern Psychiatry* (1953). In *The Interpersonal Theory of Psychiatry* (1953), Sullivan formulates anxiety as a postulate. "The tension of anxiety, when present in the mothering one, induces anxiety in the infant" (Sullivan). An infant's anxiety is a feeling state the exact nature of which one cannot specify because infants are unable to tell anyone how they feel (1953). How early in life they experience this "fear-like" state one cannot say. It has nothing to do with a hypothetical birth trauma; nor does it have anything to do with dammed up libidinal energy which, according to Freud in his earlier formulations, became converted into anxiety. For Sullivan, there are two problems about infants' experience of anxiety. First, in what sort of state or states does the mothering one induce anxiety? Second, how do anxiety states get induced? With regard to the first problem, Sullivan stressed the existence of anxiety in the mothering one, although in some of his later lectures he held that if the mothering one is disturbed (perhaps after a quarrel with her neighbor or some upsetting occurrence when she is shopping), these experiences may also induce anxiety in the infant because the mothering one may remain disturbed when she returns to the immediate environment of her offspring. Sullivan did not know, as stated above, how early in infancy an individual may experience anxiety. That is a problem for future research in which anxiety will have been clearly differentiated from fear, during infancy.

The second question is equally difficult to answer. In *Conceptions of Modern Psychiatry* (1953), Sullivan postulated the existence of an emotional contagion or communion between the infant and the mothering one. He speculated that the period of greatest importance of this emotional linkage, which he called *empathy*, is from age six to 27 months. Since Sullivan asserted that this empathic communication did not occur through ordinary sensory channels, or if it did, he did not know how, his formulation of empathy encountered a good deal of criticism after it appeared in print. In any event, Sullivan recast his formulation. The clinician in the psychiatric emergency room is well acquainted with this phenomenon, e.g. the patient who seeks help because he may "lose control" will become more anxious if the psychiatrist presents anxious responses. In that sense the therapist's anxiety is "contagious" (Melinek, 1980).

Anxiety in the mothering one *somehow* induces anxiety in her offspring. In later years, Sullivan greatly expanded his formulation of the induction of anxiety although this formulation is foreshadowed in *Conceptions of Modern Psychiatry* (1953). For example, the mothering one can "communicate" or induce feelings by the quality of facial expression, spoken language, etc. even before the infant starts learning to talk. Thus, the frowns of an anxious mother can induce a "fear-like state," anxiety in the infant. Unwittingly or wittingly the mothering one may modify her infant's behavior by "forbidding gestures" such as frowning at the baby's behavior. Analogously she can reinforce a particular behavior pattern by encouraging gestures such as smiling, patting him gently, etc.

Brazelton et al. (1974) have demonstrated in a carefully conducted investigation (with the aid of videotape microanalysis) a set of interactive behaviors which were demonstrable in optimal face to face interaction between infants and their mothers. This was characterized by a rhythm of attention-nonattention which seems to define a cyclical homeostatic curve of attention. When the mother acted inattentively, the rythmic interaction was violated and resulted in the child's distress which included an "anxiety like" behavior.

These studies seem to support Sullivan's notion about the induction of anxiety in the young infant (Brazelton et al., 1974; Tronick et al., 1975; Brazelton et al., 1975).

PERSONIFICATIONS OF THE CHILD

Since the baby's senses are not yet fully mature, and since he will take years to channel his sense experiences into useful and more or less accurate person perceptions (to say nothing of the long period required for the full maturation of the brain), the baby's perception of the mothering one will probably be for an indefinitely specifiable length of time to some degree rudimentary and unstable. In other words, the infant perceives the mother as she actually relates to him, but cannot perceive her dealings with her husband, relatives, friends, or neighbors in the way they perceive her.

Perhaps no one knew better than Sullivan the difficulties of *person perception*. In various lectures, he distinctly conveyed the belief that the "average person's" perceptions of people are profoundly flawed. Gordon Allport's book (1961) on personality has a great deal to offer regarding person perception and reveals a great many of its complexities.

The infant forms an "image," or personification of the mothering one in accordance with what *he* sees, feels, hears, smells, etc., when she feeds him, changes his wet or soiled diapers, bathes him, plays with him, etc. For the most part, in Western Society, the mothering one is the biological mother. For the sake of convenience we assume she has a husband and perhaps other children, although we know the divorce and desertion rates in the United States are formidably high. This has to be borne in mind. We are not dealing with precisely the sort of family that has existed in, for example, Italy for centuries, at least until very recently when it is losing its cohesiveness.

However, regardless of the mothering one's social situation, when she behaves tenderly and satisfies the infant's needs she is the *"good mother"* according to Sullivan. She is a being quite different (in the infant's experience) from the mothering one who is anxious and upset while nursing and caring for him. The latter induces anxiety tension, which interferes with and makes difficult sucking and swallowing milk or formula. This differently experienced mothering one, because she arouses discomfort and unwittingly makes the satisfaction of hunger or some other satisfaction on another occasion unpleasant or painful, is the *"bad"* mother. Sullivan held that a young infant, as a result of the two kinds of experiences, actually *"prehends"* or perceives in some rudimentary fashion two different beings, one is perceived as good, the other, as bad. Of course, the infant is too immature to employ such categories, but from his experiences with hundreds of patients Sullivan inferred that such a bifurcation of experience must have occurred. An infant cannot talk about satisfaction or tenderness, fear, anxiety, or pain, but he can experience them, and they apparently govern his rudimentary perceptions and behaviors up to late infancy or early childhood. There is nothing inherently mysterious about these matters. If an adult is made anxious or fearful by another person, he may soon begin to perceive the other person quite differently. Imagine how differently a young man who entered into an unsuccessful marriage perceived his wife on the day of their marriage—and again on the day of their divorce.

Today, the importance of this first interpersonal relationship is neither startling nor controversial. In fact, it has become an established conception and a starting point for thinking about what infants do. It has been accepted that the nature of our earliest relationships greatly influences the course of relations to come and "missteps in the dance" of the first interpersonal relationship as Daniel Stern (1977) coins it "the first relationship," are now considered to be of utmost developmental importance.

> If we could capture the essence of the nature of characteristic transactive patterns of any individual infant-caregiver pair, it might be possible, even feasible, to predict and chart the likely course of future interpersonal relatedness. Yet this task eludes us; both parents and researchers maintain that some temperamental features of infants, such as activity level, remain consistent during development (Thomas et al., 1963)

Furthermore, at a different level, most parents experience that the interpersonal "feel" of what it is like to be with the person who is their child maintains some indescribable yet pervasively recognizable unbroken strain from infancy on, even though the manifestations of this "feel" may change considerably during different developmental epochs. We have all experienced this in most of our long term relationships (Stern, 1977).

The notion of "bad" and "good" mother as perceived by the infant has gained new significance by current writers (Kerenberg, 1975). In this notion, as in so many other conceptions, Sullivan has proven to be a great pioneer.

MOTHER'S PERSONIFICATIONS OF THE INFANT

Because person perception is (almost) by definition one of the cornerstones of interpersonal theory, one must bear in mind that the mother's perception of her infant is by no means perfectly accurate, absolutely veridical. Her personality structure and her conceptions of her role as a mother make a reasonably accurate perception of her offspring virtually impossible. During the course of infancy and early childhood, the mother must gradually introduce relatively mild restrictions in order to discharge her social responsibilities as the "Carrier of Cultural Standards." For example, she must teach the youngster various habits, including eating, how to control and regulate defecation, urination, etc. Current research has been devoting more and more attention to the "caregiver's repertoire" as manifested by mother's baby talk (Stern, 1977), "universal facial greeting behaviors" (Eibl-Eibesfeldt, 1970), forms of vocalization and language (Snow, 1972; Lenneberg and Lenneberg, 1975), mutual gaze, etc.

Interpersonal Situations in Infancy

Of the several kinds of interpersonal situations that are inherent to the stage of infancy, we have stressed those connected with the mother's nursing and caring for the infant. The reason is that Sullivan stresses them in the organization of the personifications of mother (good mother and bad mother) which in childhood fuse into one *mother* and good and bad me's into one *me*. For the purposes of this book, one can almost ignore his discussion of the anal and urethral *zones of interaction*. They do not constitute a stage of development. Regardless of their biological importance, they are not singled out as of prime psychological importance. The same applies to the genital zones. Unless the mothering one attaches some peculiar significance to any of these zones, and communicates it to the infant, their importance can be safely taken for granted in the infant's personality development, somewhat like, for example, the "manual zone." But, if the mothering one regards any area or function of the body as disgraceful and disgusting, then that area or function becomes "marked" in a peculiar fashion. Suppose the mother or her surrogate regards "tinkering" with the anal zone or the genitals in such a fashion. Then, the youngster gradually gets the idea that such activities are to be avoided or, if he is old enough, concealed or carried on when mother is not around.

Thus, a part of the body or its peculiar functions are *not* "all right". They are bad and closely associated with anxiety, owing to the mother's attitudes or disapproval. Manual activity seems like a perfectly neutral sort of thing, incapable of arousing anxiety when the youngster employs manual skill in everyday affairs. But, let a hostile parent or parent surrogate ridicule the youngster's manual dexterity, and in a matter of months he may be "no good" with his hands.

One more illustration from a later stage will suffice to reinforce this peculiarity of some parent-child relationships. Suppose the parent tells his (or her) offspring that he is no good at spelling and laughs at his efforts. Before long, spelling will become freighted with anxiety and the child "will not be able to spell." Rubenstein and Levitt (1977) have worked with boys who were having serious difficulty in mastering routine educational tasks. In their studies, they seem to support the ideas of Sullivan. "Environmental interaction is so frustrating for these children that passivity and negation become prime resources" (Rubenstein and Levitt, 1977). The childs' energies are consumed in efforts to master his frustration in relation to the anxiety producing caretaker to the extent that his ability to learn is compromised. "The adaptive function of the ego is at the service of management of affect and is unavailable for cognitive work."

LEARNING: THE ORGANIZATION OF EXPERIENCE

During the first two years of life, maturation proceeds at a spectacular rate. But, before learning can occur, one must have appropriate and useful experience. According to Sullivan, by the end of the ninth month of infancy there are organizations of experience (visual, auditory, affective, etc.) which are manifested in recall and foresignt in many of the categories of behavior that make up the fully human type of living. Needless to say, these organizations are imperfectly developed. But the point is that they are manifested in patterns "which make it highly probable that the rudiments of a large area of human living are already organized by the end of the ninth month" (Sullivan, 1953). These organizations of behavior pertain largely, but not exclusively, to situations involving the satisfaction of needs. The first of all learning is said to be in connection with *anxiety*. From severe anxiety one learns nothing. But less severe anxiety allows for gradual realization of the situation in which it occurs. Sullivan taught that even from very early in life, at a point in time which he could not specify exactly, there is "learning of an inhibitory nature." (Watson and Skinner would say that conditioning occurs remarkably early in life.)

The next process of learning is vastly more important, since it appears to be the beginning of social learning. It is learning on the basis of what Sullivan called the "anxiety gradient"; that is, "learning to discriminate increasing from diminishing anxiety and to alter anxiety in the direction of the latter." (Sullivan 1953). This means that very early in life one learns when one is getting more anxious. The infant tinkering with the anus feels anxious when his mother is present, and "notices" that this does not occur, or at least much less painfully when he fiddles through a blanket. In some lectures, Sullivan employed the illustration of tinkering with the penis, and how, in a similar fashion, the child gradually alters his behavior to tinkering with the umbilicus. Of course, many mothers tend to keep their babies tightly diapered, at least in the United States, and, therefore, the infant's opportunities for auto-erotic behavior are limited. Still, babies do sometimes shake loose from their diapers unless the mothering one is constantly vigilant during waking hours. And constant vigilance, apart from the fact that she has many chores to take care of, can be wearing on mother.

The point of these illustrations is that very early in human life the infant unwittingly adopts some pattern of activity which will partially satisfy a need under circumstances whose complete satisfaction in a different set of circumstances entails painful anxiety. Of course, the infant cannot think about such matters and say to himself, "Ma, for some unearthly reason, doesn't like me to do this so I must find a way to outwit her." The young infant cannot deliberate. Yet, the rudiments of intelligence are already there, and he is able to discriminate the increase or decrease of anxiety and modify his behavior. This *unwitting* alteration of behavior is what Sullivan meant by *sublimation* To put this another way, there is "the long-circuiting" of the resolution of situations — a long circuiting which is socially acceptable. In the process of learning, from stage to stage, the youngster is required to sublimate a great deal, but in the beginning sublimation has only a remote connection with the customs of society or social group. It is impossible to specify how many kinds of needs are capable of sublimation, but there are some which obviously cannot be; the need for food, for water, for sleep, for the elimination of waste products, for exercise and activity at appropriate times.

The next important learning process is trial and success learning. Trial and error learning may be often defined as the process, in the face of anxiety, of attempting to solve a problem by trying out various possibilities and discarding those that are unsatisfactory. This kind of learning, although it need not relate to anxiety, is perhaps more important in everyday life than contemporary psychology texts tend to stress. In discussing *trial and success* learning in infancy, Sullivan employs a very simple illustration. It pertains to an activity that is vital to the infant: learning how to suck. This is said to be accomplished — after a number of misses — by trial movements of the extremities, aided by a certain amount of visual sentience and a good deal of kinesthetic sentience.

These experiences form the beginning distinction of "my body" in contrast to everything else. Sullivan stresses another very important instance of *trial and error learning* which appears by the sixth to the eighth month of the infant's life. This is the incipient learning of phonemes by trial and error from human example. In this fashion of trial and success learning, the infant begins to "approximate" sounds *made* by him to sounds *heard* by him. Another process of *learning* is *learning from rewards and punishments*, which begins at an undeterminately early age. The fondling or pleasure-giving manipulation of the youngster is perhaps the first. Rewards are of many kinds. Sullivan asserted that, in general, rewards take the pattern of a change from relative indifference to the offspring to more or less active interest in and approval of whatever he seems to be doing. In this manner, it appears, the need for an audience response is stamped in.

Ever since Thorndike, American psychologists have been warning their readers that punishment is likely to be not only non-educative, but psychologically harmful as well. Certainly, one can find many instances in which these views are borne out. But, it is very doubtful that these ideas are valid with regard to *parents who love their children*. Be that as it may, Sullivan disagreed with the mainstream of psychological thought regarding the role of punishment and, typically, showed that he had the courage of his convictions. With regard to late infancy he wrote,

> from then on through life, punishments are commonly the inflicting of *pain*, the refusal of contact or of attention, and of course, the inducing of anxiety—a very special punishment. I know of no reason why punishment should be undesirable as an educative influence excepting it be anxiety-ladened. Pain has a very useful function in life and loneliness and the foresight of enforced isolation, the "fear of ostracism", is bound to be an important influence from early in the third stage (the juvenile era) of development (Sullivan, 1953).

Trial and error learning from human example appears quite early, although Sullivan did not know how early. Recent research, however, suggests that such behavior patterns as facial expressions observed in newborn infants as early as one hour after birth is an innate ability of human beings, rather than the product of many months of postnatal development, as has been thought, and is based on the infants' ability to use intermodal equivalences (Melzaff and Moore, 1977; Charlesworth and Krentzer, 1973). (One should be careful not to confuse facial imitation with social smiling, which has different meanings in different cultures.)

Sullivan held that early in infancy, (mid infancy) because of contact with the mothering one and any other significant people, as previously mentioned, the infant has learned certain patterns of postural (muscular) tensions of the face that are right and wrong. Smiling is a typical example, in which there is coordination and change of posture of the face. Such a posture does not remain fixed—in an adult one can observe fairly subtle gradations of change of facial posture—because it would otherwise become a static feature. Frowning is another typical facial posture which one learns by trial and error from human example. In this fashion, a number of facial expressions are learned. They are or become important communicative devices and modes of expression. Trial and error learning from human example covers a broad field and is by no means confined to facial expression. Recent observations support and add to Sullivan's conception of a smile. Daniel Stern summarizes the current developmental approach to infants' smile in his book on "the first relationship" (Stern, 1977). The "smile" moves from a reflexive activity (internally triggered) to a species of social responses (as Sullivan conceived it) which are externally elicited by humans' (interpersonal relations) and other stimulation to instrumental behavior, to a sufficiently coordinated behavior to combine with other facial expressions.

The Acquisition of Speech

Sullivan thought that trial and error learning from human example is the chief agency in the acquisition of language. The infant learns to approximate the phonemes or "particular sound areas" that are used by the significant people around him from an indefinitely great number of vocal sounds that he utters. The significant people reinforce the "correct" sounds and sound patterns. Those sounds he utters which are not found in his parents' language disappear. Paradoxically, it is difficult to learn those sounds, or some of them, in later life if one tries to learn a foreign language. It is also by trial and error that the infant "picks up" the patterns of tonal melody in others' speech. In short, from six to nine months, the infant can repeat syllables such as "Da-da-da-da" or "Ma-ma-ma-ma." If the mother believes her offspring now knows her pet name, she may smile and coo at him or pick him up and hug him. At about one year to 15 months the infant can say a word; approximately three to five words, at 18 months.

Of itself, language would never enable one to grasp the intricate connections in nature and the marvelously complex relations between ideas. It is true that any language has a very complex structure, which Sullivan and the linguistic anthropologist Edward Sapir (1929) (from whom Sullivan learned a good deal about language and communication) thought is purely cultural, that is, learned. But language, whether spoken or written, does not apparently of itself bestow the priceless gift which is central to intelligence, what Spearman (1923) called the *education of relations*. Leaving aside those whose nervous system has suffered horrendous psychological trauma in early life, everyone appears to manifest a considerable degree of linguistic capability which enables people infinitely more than any other particular acquired skill to cope with the world. Of course, this capability requires not only maturation but a good deal of general and particular learning experiences. Intense anxiety can confuse one's capabilities to grasp connections in nature or relations between ideas. This great obstacle may or may not be related to cultural limitations or taboos. For example a very intelligent child may induce severe anxiety in a parent because he cannot deal with the child's persistent questioning. Therefore, the latter's curiosity becomes dulled after a time, since he cannot cope with the parent's overt disapproval. Sullivan's approach to language acquisition has recently received reinforcement from Katherine Nelson's description of the roots of language acquisition in which she underlines the importance of interpersonal functions (specifically early interpersonal nonverbal communication forms) in the emergence of speech (Nelson, 1977).

THE BEGINNINGS OF THE SELF SYSTEM

The *awareness* of the infant is thought to be of a very diffuse and unspecified kind. It would be a great mistake to confuse it with the *consciousness* of a grown up. The young infant does not *know* that he is hungry or anxious or in pain. His awareness is much too primitive for that. Only gradually does he catch on to the fact that his body is separate from everything else. Sullivan held that the relatively invariant coincidence of felt need, with foresight of satisfaction by adequate and appropriate activity, such as sucking, and with the dimly perceived or "prehended" cooperation of the mothering one in security and satisfaction, all gradually develop into a master pattern of experience which ultimately gets to be identified as "my body"—the organic anchorage of the self. During roughly the first year and a half, the infant receives what Allport called a constant stream of sensations from the internal organs of the body; from muscles, joints, tendons etc. Of course, numerous "external" sensations are also experienced, due to the fact that various events in the world impinge on the infant sense organs. Moreover, the relative passivity of early infancy gives way to increasing activity in the infant's life space. And this activity also helps to acquaint the youngster with the world and with his own body. But, Sullivan thought that the recurrent interpersonal experiences, which the infant has, provide definition, or meaning to the awareness of the body. Once an awarenes of "my body" develops it becomes an internal anchorage of the self. But, one must take care not to read into the infantile mind the consciousness (perceptions) of "my body" which adults possess.

However, it is not enough to say that interpersonal experiences covering the long stretch of what Piaget called the sensorimotor stage, the first 18 months, when there is no mediating self between sensations, feelings, and activities, provide a master pattern which gradually "teaches" the infant or prepares and enables him to "learn" what his sensations, feelings, and activities mean. It is not enough to say that interpersonal experiences largely provide the master plan or organization which welds the recurrent sensations, feelings, and activities into a coherent foundation for the self—that is, the bodily "me" forming anchorage points for the organization of the self. There is one other vital factor which has not been singled out as central to the growth of the self, even though it has been discussed in several contexts. That factor is *anxiety*.

According to Sullivan, when the infant reaches the phase where he is considered capable of *learning* (a point traditionally defined by the parents' cultural milieu), the mothering one, who is ordinarily the biological mother, increasingly modifies the exhibition of tenderness toward her infant. She restricts her tenderness, on numerous occasions, in connection with her efforts to teach her offspring various socially correct or acceptable behavior patterns. This includes the learning of various habits with regard to eating, drinking, elimination of waste products, and as time goes on, dressing, etc. The mother rewards the infant when he is good and conforms as best he can to her wishes, and withholds tenderness when he is bad. The infant is said to learn to chart his course by mild forbidding gestures (that is, occasions when mother frowns, speaks sharply and the like) or by mild states of worry or disapproval manifested by the mothering one. One might say that the "great way" of learning in infancy is by the grading of felt anxiety. This occurrence is not confined to infancy, however.

Sullivan claimed that anxiety, in its most severe form, is a rare experience after infancy in the more fortunate courses of personality development. He also held that in a highly civilized society or community confronted by no particular crisis, anxiety is never very severe for most people in a chronologically adult life. Neverless, he repeatedly asserted that it is anxiety which is responsible for a great part of the inadequate, inefficient, unduly rigid, or otherwise unfortunate performances of people. There can hardly be any doubt that a majority of people do not value themselves adequately, a condition that is marked by feelings of inferiority, lack of initiative, and a wavering self-esteem. In *Personal Psychopathology* Sullivan wrote that the "adaptive culture" of American Society is gravely deficient, lagging far behind the great advances in material culture. In the United States, it is the parents who normally introduce their offspring to the most basic features of adaptive culture, and this, in turn, tends to govern the "training" of children until they reach the fifth or sixth year. But, we do not wish to leave the impression that teaching, at any level of education, is governed by reason and sweetness and light. Teachers possess technical knowledge and various skills, but there is no evidence that they possess wisdom. It is only fair to add that mass education does not — and cannot — aim at wisdom.

Anxiety, "in a basic sense," is responsible for a great many of the problems with which a psychiatrist deals when he interviews patients. However, anxiety is not the "motor" or efficient cause of interpersonal relations. Sullivan, nevertheless, explicity states that it *more or less directs the course of their development.* It is chiefly anxiety, not the repression of sexual satisfactions, as it is experienced in various contexts, which limits or distorts normal development and hinders or precludes healthy interpersonal relations of chronological adults.

It is the role of anxiety in the development of the self-system or self dynamism with which this text is presently concerned. There are many problems connected with the self which transcend the scope of this book. Two profound chapters on the self in William James' *Principles of Psychology* (1907), or Gordon Allport's *Pattern and Growth in Personality* (1961), which enlarges upon almost every aspect of the self, can supplement the outline of self development in this book. However, there can be no question of the originality of Sullivan's formulations, whatever his debt to certain predecessors, notably the sociologist Charles Horton Cooley, William James, and the philosopher George Herbert Mead may have been.

There are two main aspects of the self, conceived from a Sullivan point of view, "good me" and "bad me," which constitute the personified self, which is part of the self-system, a formation which has often given readers of Sullivan considerable trouble. Because he attempted to trace the origins of the self-system (or self) back to infancy, Sullivan states, *in the language of adults*, what he believes *must have occurred* first during infancy and early childhood. As Sullivan states:

> From experience of these three sorts (the third is "not me" — or part of the dissociated) with rewards, with the anxiety—there comes an initial personification of three phases of what will presently be *me*, that which is invariably connected with the sentience of *my* body—and you will remember that *my* body as an organization of experience has come to be distinguished from everything else by its self-sentient character (Sullivan, 1972).

These three sorts of beginning personifications are organized in about mid-infancy. The thing that always keeps them in close connection, binding them ultimately into one, is their relatedness to the growing conception of "my body."

At the risk of laboring what may seem obvious—although it is always risky to assume anything in Sullivan is obvious, "good-me" and "bad-me" will be reviewed, followed by explicate "bad-me." First of all, there is no one-to-one correspondence between the infant's personifications of his mother and his growing personifications of himself. So, a review of "good-me" and "bad-me" will serve as a precautionary measure, since for many years the subtleties of Sullivanian psychology have proven to be a grave obstacle to the understanding of interpersonal psychiatry. In the exposition of interpersonal theory, it is best to let Sullivan speak for himself, as it were, on the topic of the self.

> *Good-me* is the beginning personification which organizes experience in which satisfactions have been enhanced by rewarding increments of tenderness, which come to the infant because the mothering one is pleased with the way things are going; therefore, and to that extent, she is free, and moves toward expressing tender appreciation of the infant. Good-me, as it ultimately develops, is the ordinary topic of discussion (Sullivan, 1972).

This, in capsule form, is how the experience of self-esteem starts, although subsequent unfortunate experience may undermine it.

> *Bad-me*, on the other hand, is the beginning personification which organizes experience in which increasing degrees of anxiety are associated with behavior involving the mother one in its more-or-less clearly prehended interpersonal setting (Sullivan, 1972).

Prehension is the most rudimentary form of perception. In early infancy, it is not very far along the sensation-perception spectrum of experience, because the infant's awareness is well below the level of consciousness. Perception provides information or misinformation readily accessible to consciousness. Thus, .the nipple-in-lips experience is one form of sentience. Sentience provides the starting point for obtaining information.

As maturation and sensory experience proceed all through infancy, the youngster approaches the capability to perceive an object or event. Even in early childhood, the youngster's perceptions are relatively rudimentary. Speech, as it is acquired, is a mighty aid in the act of perceiving. The frequent coincidence of certain behavior on the part of the infant — some of which has been previously discussed — with increasing tension and increasingly evident forbidding on the part of the mother is said to be the source of the type of experience which is organized as the rudimentary personification, "bad-me." But "bad-me" in the course of development becomes definitely a part of the self-system.

Not-me (not of me) is manifested in dissociated behavior, which is perhaps most clearly evident in every day life "absences" (of consciousness) or in "naturally occurring trance states" (Spiegel and Spiegel, 1978) and at times in "grave mental disorders" such as severe schizophrenic episode or dissociative disorders such as Psychogenic Amnesia, Psychogenic Fugue, Multiple Personality, etc. (as described in DSM III [American Psychiatric Association, 1979]).

Even when dissociation "works," it works very suavely, acording to Sullivan. It works by a continuous alertness or vigilance of the self-system, so that any evidences of dissociated processes are selectively inattended.

Selective inattention, a process which makes it possible not to notice almost "an infinite series of more or less meaningful details of one's living" is employed. This is seemingly most conspicuous in obsessive-compulsive neuroses. Most of us usually encounter the operation of "not-me" processes in a nightmare. When one wakes up after a nightmare, one may not know who he is or where he is. Perhaps, for a few seconds, one can recall intensely terrifying events of the dream process. Ordinarily, it is inexplicable and incommunicable. Normally, the self intervenes swiftly and one very quickly regains his usual state of consciousness.

The rudimentary personification of "not-me" is said to evolve very gradually, since it grows from intense, recurrent, prolonged experiences of anxiety. For example, during infancy a youngster may engage in behavior which, when observed, led to intense forbidding gestures, such as scowls, frowns, expressions of embarrassment or certain tones of voice on the part of the mother or her surrogate, inducing intense anxiety in him (or her). When one suffers intense anxiety, one cannot make any sense of what has been happening. Hence, one does not know what is wrong or what to do. According to Sullivan, in later childhood, the basis provided by the "not-me" sort of experiences of early childhood may either grow or may remain more or less stationary, depending on the youngster's experiences at that time. (More of Sullivan's ideas on dissociation will be brought in as an exposition of the various phases of personality development are outlined, stage by stage.) However, in the later phase of childhood "of more fated" people who, for instance, lose a parent in childhood and get instead a very bad imitation, or are sent to an inferior institution, or something like that, there may begin to be very clear evidences of this exceedingly important system of processes to which we refer as dissociation (Sullivan, 1972).

The "not-me" component in adults is not infantile. The intensely anxiety provoking experiences of infancy and childhood which are, or become dissociated, develop, however slowly, to some extent. They change, however, slowly, as Sullivan asserted in various contexts--so slowly, perhaps that they may seem to be "stationary." He also claimed that dissociated processes persist throughout life and are manifested in various contexts. There are then two dynamic "systems" in the personality: the Self and the Dissociated. The latter is roughly analogous to the "deep unconscious" of Freudian psychology, although dissociated processes are always acquired.

Fusion of Good and Bad Mother

Sullivan claimed that during the latter part of infancy there is some evidence that the previously disperate personification of the good mother and the bad mother are never becoming fused into one personification. But, in early childhood and thereafter, the fusion is normally completed. However, in certain psychotic states the disperate personification is clearly evident. Contemporary psychiatry focuses on the problem of the borderline personality organization in which often the good and bad mother personifications are not well fused. (See Kerenberg, 1975).

THE GROWTH OF THE SELF-SYSTEM

It is from the essential desirability of being "good-me," and from the increasing ability to be warned by slight increases of anxiety in situations involving the mothering one, that the self-system comes into being. The latter is purely the product of interpersonal relations arising from anxiety encountered in the pursuit of the satisfaction of needs. Thus, it is the *anxiety gradient* —the experiences of whether one is getting more or less anxious—that is the basic influence which determines the course of interpersonal relations, and more or less directs the course of their development. More simply, the self is an organization of educative experience called into being by the necessity to avoid or minimize anxiety, or, in other words, the mother's forbidding gestures which are refinements in the personification of the bad mother. The refined discrimination of forbidding gestures first applies to the mother, the significant other person in the infant's life, and thereafter applies to practically all significant people throughout life. This phenomenon can be elaborated as follows:

> The discrimination of heard differences in the mother's face, and perhaps later of differences in speed and rhythm of her gross bodily movements in coming toward the infant, presenting the bottle, changing the diapers, or what not—all these rather refined discriminations by the distance receptors of vision and hearing are organized as indices associated with the unpleasant experience of anxiety (Sullivan, 1972).

The refinement of discrimination of *forbidding gestures* may, to some degree, continue for years, long after the real mother is firmly perceived. For example, slight changes in pitch or enunciation, a slight lifting of the eyebrow, an "awkward silence," as in the case of the mother who abruptly stops talking, can be very communicative to a child or a juvenile. In fact, many adults seem to have a repertory of forbidding and encouraging gestures.

In general, Sullivan attributes the use of forbidding gestures to the mother's necessity to "train" the child, to educate him in the employment of widespread uniformities of habits. This begins before the infant can begin to talk or understand much of what is happening to him. But, it does not follow that the mother is always conscious of the "meaning" of her forbidding gestures. She is a "carrier" of cultural norms. Therefore, she must "train" her offspring if he is to have a chance to develop into a normal human being as her society conceives normality. Ideally, she would employ forbidding gestures only for such purposes and always at appropriate times. But no one is as rational or all-knowing as that. As we have seen mothers employ forbidding gestures which are of no use to the infant, either due to his immaturity or his mother's. But a tender, loving mother, within the permissible limits imposed by her culture, is not likely to subject her offspring to much severe, recurrent anxiety. Traditionally, the caring of the offspring occurred within a firmly established and relatively secure family structure. Broken homes are apparently a more and more frequent occurrence, however. Usually, the ones who suffer most in such cases are the helpless and terribly vulnerable offspring.

As previously mentioned, in late infancy and early childhood, "good-me" and "bad-me" begin to fuse into one organization variously characterized as the self, self-system or "self-dynamism." The meaning of this is summarized by Sullivan in one brief paragraph:

> The *self-system* is a product of educative experience, part of which is of the character of reward, and a very important part of which has the graded anxiety element that we have spoken of. But quite early in life, anxiety is also a very conspicuous aspect of the self-dynamism *function*. This is another way of saying that experience functions in both recall and foresight. Since troublesome experience, organized in the self-system, has been experience connected with increasing grades of anxiety, it is not astounding that this element of recall, functioning on a broad scale, makes the intervention of the self-dynamism in living tantamount to the warning, or foresight of anxiety. And warning of anxiety or anxiety means noticeable anxiety, really a warning that anxiety will get worse (Sullivan, 1972).

All through life, the self employs a strategem called *selective inattention* which can be, and often is, employed by the person to regard anxiety-provoking occurrences and experiences as if they did not exist. If one's self-esteem is fragile, owing to a great deal of unfortunate, anxiety-provoking experience, then the use (or misuse) of selective inattention can have serious or disastrous consequences. The normal person, the individual whose experiences have been connected with recurrent tender behavior by the mother and other significant people who affect his living, learns to deal with anxiety-provoking circumstances suavely, or diplomatically. One catches on to the possibility of trouble if he does not alter his behavior or employ some technique which may mollify the other one, such as propitiatory behavior, of which there are many kinds. Unfortunately, living in an urban society is so complex that one must learn a considerable number of interpersonal skills if he is to have a fair chance for success in interpersonal relations. In addition, one should never forget that his living is always limited, if not governed, by a circumambient socio-cultural structure. In a totalitarian society, the individual's interpersonal relations are closely scrutinized and circumscribed.

There is a final point about the self which many have failed to understand. When we think of "I" or "Me," we normally think of "good-me." For obvious reasons, there is an essential desirability of living "good-me," although its infantile origins usually have been outgrown as the self-dynamism develops over the years. Normally, we shrink from the thought that at times we are objectively "bad:" aggressive, egocentric, perhaps cruelly indifferent to the feelings of others. Hence, when we think of ourselves, we tend to think of "good-me," although we can scarcely ignore the consequences and behavior of "bad-me" entirely. The fusion of "good-me" and "bad-me" is rarely, if ever, perfect. This is particularly evident in people who are insecure and lacking or limited in self-esteem, so that the feeling of "bad-me" is prominent.

In a somewhat oversimplified although nevertheless cogent exposition, Sullivan has pulled together certain limitations of the self owing to the organization it acquires, to a large degree, in early life: "The peculiarity of the self-dynamism is that as it grows it functions, in accordance with its state of development, right from the start . . . . Since the approbation of the important person is very valuable, since disapprobation denies satisfaction and give anxiety, the self becomes extremely important. It permits a minute focus on those performances of the child which are the cause of approbation and disapprobation, but, very much like a microscope, it interferes with noticing the rest of the world" (1953). In the years subsequent to the delivery of the *Conceptions* Sullivan refined this idea of the self but not to any great degree.

PERSONIFIED SELF

When a person is born, he normally has all the potentialities of becoming a full human being. But, it requires roughly 15 to 20 years before he becomes fully human. There is no convenient cut-off point where one can say a person has achieved or realized his potentialities. Sullivan, like others, has taught that the newborn human animal takes many years to acquire the attributes or characteristics which will make him a person, a human being, however imperfect. To put this in more exact Sullivan phraseology, it takes 15 or more years for the newborn infant to acquire a mature personality, which includes the Self and the Dissociated. Usually one thinks of himself as "I" or "Me." But, this is not the self. It is the personified self, which is a "quasi-entity." The self-system includes much more. For example, it includes characteristics that we have selectively inattended.

Since selective inattention is very important in Sullivan theory, its meaning must be emphasized. Attention is selective. We normally focus on certain objects or events that are significant to the understanding of some problem and ignore the rest. However, if one is or becomes anxious, he may not notice or at least perceive *relevant* aspects of a problematic situation. If one is compelled to misuse selective inattention in this fashion daily, he will fail to learn many things he should know. One is tempted to paraphrase Santayana to the effect that if one cannot learn from one's personal mistakes, one is doomed to repeat them. In any case, if one is compelled to resort to such a formidable hindrance to learning as selective inattention in various recurrent interpersonal situations, he is doomed to miss a great deal that is necessary for successful or contented living.

Thus, the personified self (sometimes ambiguously called the self-concept) is never synonymous with the self-system. We may feel things, say things, do things, even fantasize about them without ever knowing what their meaning is. Unfortunately, perhaps no one is completely free of the misuse of selective inattention.

Several times the term *dynamism*, as in self-dynamism, has been used in contrast to Freud's use of "mechanism." First of all, the smallest useful abstraction which can be employed in the functional activity of the organism itself is said to be a dynamism, just as the cell is ordinarily the smallest useful abstraction in elementary biology. By dynamism Sullivan says he means "the relatively enduring pattern of energy transformations which recurrently characterize the organism in its duration as a living organism." If matter and energy are conventible, the definition has a serious flaw. Thoughts do not have mass—a basic characteristic of matter.

However, such technical difficulties must not lead us astray. A biologist who is studying an organ or organ system, unless some special inquiry requires it, ordinarily ignores the fact that the smallest functional unit is the cell. Analogously, in this book, we will ignore the fact that, emotions, motivations, sensations are hierarchies of "dynamisms." There is the further consideration that it is difficult to understand how thoughts (which often are of brief duration) passing through a person's mind are "dynamisms," unless one conceives thoughts as mere neurophysiological occurrences—a questionable assumption. At the present time, people either ignore this problem or equate mind and brain. Regardless of current ideas, we adhere to the traditional view that man thinks. This is an axiom to be accepted, not to be proved.

Although the logical difficulty mentioned above remains, the following quotation will, serve our purposes in this book:

> The dynamisms of interest to the psychiatrist are the relatively enduring patterns of energy transformation which recurrently characterize the interpersonal relations—the functional interplay of persons and personifications, personal signs, personal abstractions, and personal attributions—which make up the distinctively human sort of being (Sullivan, 1972).

REFERENCES

Allport, G. *Pattern and Growth in Personality.* Holt, Rinehart and Winston, New York, 1961.

American Psychiatric Association, Task Force on Nomenclature and Statistics. *DSM III –Diagnostic and Statistical Manual of Mental Disorders*, Third ed. Washington, D.C., APA, 1979.

Brenner, C. *An Elementary Textbook of Psychoanalysis*. Doubleday, New York, 1955.

Brazelton, T. B., Koslowski, B., and Main, M. "The Origins of Reciprocity in Mother-Infant Interaction," in Lewis, M., and Rosenblum, L.A. eds., *The Effect of the Infant on Its Caregiver*. Wiley-Interscience, New York, 1974.

Brazelton, T. B., Tronick, E., Adamson, L., Als, H., and Wise, S. "Early Mother-Infant Reciprocity," in *Parent-Infant Interaction*. Ciba Foundation Symposium 33, 1975.

Charlesworth, W. R., and Krentzer, M. "Facial Expressions of Infants and Children," in Ekman, P. ed., *Darwin and Facial Expression*. Academic Press, New York, 1973.

Ciba Foundation Symposium. *Discussion on Qualities of Relationships: Parent-Infant Interaction*. M. Hoffer, chairman, 1975.

Eibl-Eibesfeldt, I. *Ethology, The Biology of Behavior*. Holt, Rinehart and Winston, New York, 1970.

Eriksen, E. *Childhood and Society*. W.W. Norton, New York, 1950.

Freud, S. *New Introductory Lectures on Psychoanalysis*. W. W. Norton, New York, 1949.

James, W. *The Principles of Psychology*, 2 vols. Henry Holt, New York, 1907.

Kerenberg, O. *Borderline Conditions and Pathological Narcissism*. Jason Aronson, Inc., New York, 1975.

Lenneberg, E. and Lenneberg, E. eds. *Foundations of Language Development I*. Academic Press, New York, 1975.

Linn, L. Diagnosis and Psychiatry, Symptoms of Psychiatric Disorders, in Freedman, A. M., Kaplan, H. C. and Sadak, B. S. eds., *Comprehensive Textbook of Psychiatry III*. Williams and Wilkins, Baltimore, 1980.

Melinek, M. *The angry violent patient*. Emergency Med. Series of Southern Med. Assoc. Dial Access Syst., 1980.

Melzaff, A. N., and Moore, M. K. Imitation of facial and manual gestures by human neonates. *Science*. 1977; 198: 75.

Nelson, K. First steps in language acquisition. *J. Am. Acad. Child Psychiat.* 1977; 16: 563–583.

Quadagno, D. M., McCollough, J., Ho, G. K., and Spevak, H. M. Neonatal bonadal hormones: Effect on maternal behavior and sexual behavior in the female rat. *Physiol. Behav.* 1973; 11: 231–254.

Rubenstein, B., and Levitt, M. Learning disabilities as related to a special form of mothering. *J. Psychoanal.* 1977; 58: 45–55.

Sapir, E. The status of linguistics as a science. *Language*. 1929; 5: 207–214.

Sartain, A. Q., North A. J., Strange, J. R., and Chapman, H. M. *Psychology: Understanding Human Behavior*. McGraw-Hill, New York, 1973.

Snow, C. Mother's speech to children learning language. *Child Dev.* 1972; 43: 549–564.

Spearman, C. *The Nature of "Intelligence" and the Principles of Cognition*. Macmillan, New York, 1923.

Spiegel, H., and Spiegel, D. *Trance and Treatment*. Basic Books, New York, 1978.

Stern, D. *The First Relationship*. Harvard University Press, Cambridge, 1977.

Sullivan, H. S. *Conceptions of Modern Psychiatry*. W. W. Norton, New York, 1953.

Sullivan, H. S. *The Interpersonal Theory of Psychiatry*. W. W. Norton, New York, 1953.

Sullivan, H.S. *Personal Psychopathology*. W.W. Norton, New York, 1972.

Thomas, A., Birch, H. G., Chess, S., Hertzig, M. E. and Korn, S. *Behavioral Individuality in Early Childhood*. New York University Press, New York, 1963.

Tronick, E., Adamson, L., Wise, S., Als, H., and Brazelton, T. B. "Mother-Infant Face-to-Face Interaction," in Gosh, S. ed., *Biology and Language*. Academic Press, London, 1975.

3

The Transition from Infancy

There is no day, week, or even month at which one can say that all babies begin to walk. For several reasons, infants begin to walk at different ages. The "average" is 15 months. It is the same thing with talking. There is no one definite month when all babies start talking. This also applies to a great many other occurrences in infancy and childhood. That is why it is safer and more accurate to distinguish stages, epochs, or eras of development. Then, in normal situations, one can say the offspring develops certain skills, during this or that era. Even then, as development proceeds, one must allow for considerable individual differences. One should also allow for differences due to cultural requirements, but this exceeds the scope of this book. If one is curious about some of the differences which are due to cultural factors in societies that are vastly different from American society, he might read some of the works of the ever-popular Margaret Mead or Ruth Benedict.

One must realize that definitions, classifications, and various other logical tools exist for a purpose. In the natural and social sciences, they foster inquiry and contribute to the solution of practical problems, which often furthers inquiry. For reasons that will presently be made clear Sullivan thought that during the course of personality development, certain critical capabilities normally appear at each phase of development. He also thought that no one can leap over a given phase and proceed headlong toward maturity. It seems that human capabilities appear in a fairly orderly sequence, given the appropriate kind of environment. If some of them are not developed, they may be very difficult — sometimes impossible — to develop later on even under prolonged intensive psychotherapy.

Partly because Sullivan believed language and communication, (which itself may be considered a form of language), are such a transcendentally important dimension of culture, he distinguished the first era — infancy, from the next era, childhood, the ability to utter articulate sounds of or pertaining to speech, is outstanding up to the next phase when the youngster manifests the need for playmates, the *juvenile* era.

However, one phase blends gradually into the next. Thus, there is a transitional phase from infancy to childhood during which much previous learning—both fortunate and unfortunate—becomes consolidated, while new capabilities begin to appear. Some illustrations may help. It has been pointed out that during late infancy parents, especially the mothering one, increase their efforts to socialize the infant, that is, to teach him or enable him to learn various habits that are essential, not only to future development, but to living in a given community or society. Once more, we will avail ourselves of a formulation from Gordon Allport's classic work. He wrote:

> Think for a moment of how many *kinds* of learning take place in the course of life. We learn to walk, talk, and dance; to drive automobiles, swim and play the piano; to spell, write and read; we memorize facts, phone numbers, and poems. We learn what to eat, what to fear, what to shun and what objects to desire sexually. We acquire morals, values, and interests. We come to embrace religions, beliefs, ideologies. We develop preferences, prejudices, and manners. We learn new concepts, meanings and conformities; also foreign languages. We learn new motives, ambitions, and hopes. We learn signs, cues, and symbols. Gradually we acquire our own traits and trends of personality...(Allport, 1961).

Much of the learning which Allport has summarized has been mainly acquired outside the home, which provides a scaffolding for most human learning.

In the socializing, humanizing process, the element of frequency in the infant's experience as he proceeds to learn more and more complex activities is vital. So is consistency—the repetition of a particular pattern of events. It follows that inconsistencies in the efforts of the parent can have grave consequences. Sullivan was not too sure when inconsistency begins to undermine profitable learning. He said that many of the difficulties which manifest themselves from the end of the first year onward may prove to be the accumulating results of inconsistencies in the efforts of the acculturating parent. Current research provides more information on this subject that confirms Sullivan's uncanny ability to understand infancy. The importance of consistency, inconsistency, sequential behavior, structure and timing of behavior or what Daniel Stern (1977) calls "the repetitive run" has been proven to be of utmost importance in infant's development. When the child is using speech as his outstanding acquisition around the third year of life, the extent to which the parent fails to provide a relatively invariant pattern of responses takes on great significance.

LACK OF SANITY OF THE EDUCATIONAL EFFORT

Sullivan regarded certain of the mother's educational efforts as "insane," such as treating a one-year-old baby as if he were willfully troublesome, trying to teach him to be clean and dry when he is only 15 months old, restricting the freedom of the infant's manual explorations after his accidental discovery that the external genitals are a source of keen sentience so that he becomes fearfully upset, etc. Such efforts not only are the source of intense anxiety—for example, in connection with the last illustration, in later life the youngster may develop various peculiarities about the use of the genitals—but they also interfere with the infant's budding maturation of the capacity for observation, exploration, and elaboration of experience at a given time. Still again, one must mention the type of mother who regrets that the infant must grow up and encourages him to "stay put." Working against the process of maturation, she provides rewards and arouses anxiety (due to disapproval) in her offspring which are designed to try to keep the infant or child young.

This kind of not "letting go or grow" is fairly common, especially in later life when children are expected in our society to leave home, or act more independently. The fear of the "empty nest" may lead parents to develop mental or physical symptoms which may prevent the offspring from leaving home. The following example will illuminate this point: An 18-year-old female who was brought to the Emergency Room of a hospital was suffering from an overdose of tranquilizers and was accompanied by her crippled mother. In the interview following the patient's revival, she presented severe depression related to her having been forbidden by her mother to attend a college far from home. It seems that when the mother learned about her daughter's intention of leaving home, she developed a severe back pain with difficulties in walking which was not helped by the effort of numerous physicians and therefore, forced her daughter to stay home and take care of her.

OVERT AND COVERT PROCESSES

Sullivan claimed that up to the ninth or tenth month, the observer must rely on inference in connection with certain infantile experience. It is not subject to clear, objective demonstration. One can only infer with some—perhaps considerable—probability of correctness as to what sort of experiences the infant had from what can be observed. This leads to a distinction which is likely to be familiar to the reader—the distinction between overt processes in interpersonal relations and covert processes. For example, a baby may manifest various signs of being disturbed when the telephone rings. His face may become red, while he yells and thrashes about in his crib. He may even point to the ringing telephone. A devoted parent may wonder, as he observes such phenomena, what is occurring in the infant's mind. The answer may be jealousy; this is an inference. Since jealous behavior has also been observed even in baby animals, it seems to be a probably correct inference. This inference may be strengthened if a year or two later, the child continues to show what is then unmistakable evidence of jealousy.

In connection with covert processes, one can infer the existence of *delayed behavior*, especially during the latter months of infancy. It seems to be well established that needs have a hierarchical organization. An observer may note that sometimes hunger may take precedence over something else that is going on, and behavior directed toward the satisfaction of hunger may interrupt whatever was occurring up to that point. (If one wished to be very rigorous he might, as per Skinner, define hunger in terms of the number of hours which elapse between feeding times). After the hunger has been satisfied, the baby may resume the interrupted activity. Sullivan asserted that, occasionally, when the interrupted activity is resumed, there has been some change in the situational pattern. It is not implausible to infer that something occurred in connection with the interrupted activity, while the covert process of satisfying hunger proceeded vigorously. Since infants have minds, regardless of what some parents may believe, it is not reckless to assume that the intervening, unseen process was mental in charater. However, it would be silly to attribute the mental abilities of an adult to an infant or child. In fact, many covert processes which are acceptable at age 12 months have to be rigidly excluded from consciousness subsequently as the self develops, chiefly owing to learning under the guidance of anxiety.

THE LEARNING OF GESTURE AND LANGUAGE

From the end of the first year onward, one learns various types of gesture and language. The perfecting of these requires months and years. Traditionally, those who have been brought up in the "Anglo-Saxon" culture or its American variant tend to use expressive gestures with reserve. But, gestures like language, may communicate thought as well as feeling. Hence, one must be alert to the context in which Sullivan employs "gesture." The learning of facial gestures is largely accomplished by trial and error from human example. No infant is born with a "poker face" or the capability to employ a "withering" or disdainful expression. No infant, according to Sullivan, is born with the ability to smile, although he manifests grimaces which can be wrongly interpreted as smiles or frowns. The adults who are frequently or generally in the company of the youngster become models from whom he learns. For this reason, a Japanese smile is very different from that of an American. Analogously, one may learn to use one's hands and arms as gestures, as is markedly the case with first generation Italians. Americans shake hands or, on occasion clap hands, but they tend to disdain the rich repertory of bodily gestures possessed by the Italians. There is reason to believe that girls usually possess much more finesse in the use of gestures than do males. Some girls have been known to practice facial expressions — and possibly other sorts of gestures — in front of a mirror. Meanwhile, their brothers may be out on the athletic field practicing baseball or football.

The learning of verbal pantomime occurs well before the twelfth month — again to a large degree by trial and error from human example. Sullivan (1956) mentions an infant he observed, who was 10 or 11 months of age and who "was carrying on a very interesting conversation of his own." Sullivan said,

> I discovered that what had caught my attention was the beautiful tonal pattern. Only perhaps 50 percent of the sounds were, I would say, good phonemal stations in the English language, but the melody, the pattern of tone, was speech; it was what our speech would be like if speech were not articulate.

However, because the infant's home was "very vocal," one has to allow for that. One cannot assume from this one illustration that infants generally acquire the melodic progression of speech by the time they have reached the eleventh or twelfth month. The reader who has struggled with the melodic progression of speech while trying to learn French or German in high school can perhaps better appreciate how much the infant has learned by the time he has reached the age of 18 months. Thus, even before the era of childhood, the infant "picks up" more and more of the non-verbal although communicative aspects of speech behavior. The first of these, according to Sullivan, is the progression of tones and silences; the rhythmic tonal pattern of the mothering one's language. One must emphasize that silence is very much a part of speech. There are many instances when we encounter "dead silence" as a response.

Sullivan's observations have been supported by contemporary students of the evolution of the language of the child such as Snow (1972) and Slobin (1975) who studied "*How* the mother talks rather than what she says." Another fascinating classic paper by Ferguson (1964) made it clear that what Sullivan refers to in the quotation mentioned above is valid all over the world.

There is another aspect to the learning of language which cannot be ignored: the responses of the mother and other significant people, such as the father and older siblings. This point has already been brought up, but it deserves reiteration. When the infant of eight or nine months, who is already learning the melodic progression of his parents' language, happens to utter a string of sounds such as da-da-da and ma-ma-ma at an appropriate time, an enthusiastic parent may get the idea that the infant has learned the pet names of the parents, or at least one of the parents. It may happen that mother suspects or wants to believe that her infant has learned her pet name. Let us assume that on such occasions mother picks up her infant and hugs him or kisses him. In short, she acts tenderly toward him in some fashion familiar to parents. What is to the infant mere repetitive syllabic experimentation from time to time approximates, at least to the mother, what used to be called baby talk. Usually this so-called baby talk gets reinforced. It arouses mother's attention, perhaps frequently tender responses, and perhaps encouragement, such as "say mama, mama" and perhaps "dada, dada." Of course, the mothering one does not stop with pet names. Gradually, she may encourage him in his use of other "words." The point is that the learning of correct speech, stretching over a period of months and years is due to trial and error learning, and trial and success encouragement and reinforcement of one sort or another. But, it is baby talk that at first generally gets stamped in. However, the stamping in of baby talk is at best only a starting point in the acquisition of language. Baby talk is not language in the usual sense of the word. The following is a more exact formulation:

> When the learning has progressed to the point where different syllabic forms, different combinations of phonemes, and some vague attempts to imitate what is heard get said, there actually appears the beginning of the extremely rich development of sounds, tonal patterns, rhythms, and what not that make up the various great and small languages of the world, including the baby's private language. It is at this time when the baby is saying things other than mere dada's and caca's and mama's, that the element of learning by reward enters in, so that the child's satisfaction in making vocal noises and hitting, by trial and error, on things that he has heard is now augmented by the tenderness of the mothering one (Sullivan, 1953).

Teaching by indifference performs an important function in the learning of the baby's language. A great many of his vocalizations do not receive any response from anyone. And so they tend to drop out of his vocal repertory because they are met with indifference. Sullivan claims that perhaps from the twelfth to the eighteenth month, to an extraordinary degree, such vocal efforts, because they do not hit the right phonemal stations in the presence of the mothering one fail of frequent repetition.

Ostracism

As interpersonal relations develop phase by phase, indifference becomes a powerful instrument of socialization. This experience of frequent or chronic indifference becomes a paradigm of the fear of ostracism. At the United States Military Academy at West Point there existed until recently a form of punishment imposed by a select group of cadets called the Honor Committee which "silenced" (socially ostracized) a cadet who had been found cheating, stealing, or lying. But, social ostracism is an ancient custom which almost always was a very effective form of punishment, sometimes amounting to death.

Autistic Language

Roughly from the twelfth to the eighteenth month, the beginnings of what Sullivan called *autistic* language, which is a species of the parataxic mode, also develops. By and large, autistic language has no communicative power. Yet, none of us, perhaps, is entirely free of autistic fringes to many of the words we use. In fact, one can point to the rather widespread use of autistic language by many people when they talk about Democracy, Justice, Property, Capitalism, etc. At any rate, the use of "words" by a youngster of 18 months has little communicative power—except perhaps to mother and father. His ability to utter a few words is no evidence that they have any meaning outside his very circumscribed life space, and not by any means always in it. But, this is a matter which needs more clarification.

LANGUAGE AS SYNTAXIC EXPERIENCE

Since the language of common speech, whether spoken or written, presupposes community, the words and sentences which persons use in everyday commerce have a relatively fixed meaning. However, if the cultural background of two people speaking the same language is different, there is likely to be some misunderstanding or obscurity in what one says to the other. Even when two people of similar backgrounds talk to each other, there is no guarantee they will understand each other perfectly. The idiosyncracies of personal experience may make perfect mutual understanding virtually impossible. In any event, when a person uses words or sentences whose meaning is verified by an implicit or sometimes explicit consensus of people in his community or society, one may say he has progressed to the syntaxic mode of experience. Such consensuses do not guarantee truth, especially when people who have not been educated in the logical niceties of language are dealing with abstract subject matters. Even so, it seems fairly safe to assume that when street cleaners talk to one another they have little difficulty understanding one another; they shout rather than talk. This may also be true of automobile manufacturers or the board members of central banks.

However, things are not quite that simple. Accent, intonation, melodic progression, and pitch are also elements of speech, and they not only may contribute to misunderstanding but often mark one as odd or "different."

If the sociologists are right when they say that every society, or the members of that society, are ethnocentric, it is no wonder that a "foreigner" becomes marked by his speech alone. One of the most common mistakes in clinical psychiatry occurs when a clinician diagnoses a patient's illness as schizophrenic on the basis of the patient's failure to follow semantic and syntactic rules, defining his illness as a "thought disorder" and not taking into consideration intellectual defect or subcultural and regional conventions.

The conventional conception of thought disorder which many clinicians have been using as one of the prominent features of schizophrenia has been lately redefined in the monumental work of the DSM III (Diagnostic and Statistical Manual of Mental Disorders 3rd ed., AMA, 1980).

It is recommended that the term "thought disorder" be avoided. The more specific terms of language disorders, communication disorders, and delusions are advocated, and the definitions of these terms stress the inability to explain the oddness of the communication by intellectual defect or subcultural and regional conventions. We welcome this development, since the term "thought disorder" is not sympathetic to Sullivan's approach which stressed language and communication, and underlined the cultural aspects of communication.

Speech and Social Class

There is another point which needs to be mentioned, although it has little or no direct bearing on *syntaxic experience* in Western societies. The speech of people who belong to different social classes is quickly noticed by most people. A generation ago, it has been said, certain world-famous English novelists of humble origin, who did not speak with an upper class "accent," and who had not attended a prestigious school, did not rate socially among the British elite. With regard to interpersonal relations, this is no trivial matter. Modes of speech and dress are two potent devices by which the upper classes set themselves off from more humble people. (However, it is perfectly all right for a member of the eminent Adams family to drive around in a rusty old jalopy). When one reaches the pinnacle of social esteem, one may discard some of the trappings of the elite. However, in some Eastern societies the gulf between the social elite and the humble is so great that they may speak different languages. But, there are other factors which separate people. In India, for example, they would include ethnic origin, class, and caste, all of which may be connected with language differences.

The Origins of Syntaxic Experience

Sullivan claimed that the first unquestionable organization of experience in the syntaxic mode is in the realm of the two great genera of communicative behavior—gesture and speech. Consensually validated symbols, whose meanings are generally "shared," may be characterized as occurring in the syntaxic mode after one has largely abandoned the autistic use of words. It may be helpful to bear in mind Edward Sapir's statement (1921) to the effect that words are the elements of language which "ticket off" experience in such a fashion that words and other symbols are associated with, and delimit classes of experience, rather than single experiences themselves. For example, in the statement "John is ill," *ill* tickets off a whole group of experiences which come under the general heading of illness. Otherwise, we would not know what the statement means.

In its most primitive meaning, consensual validation is fairly simple. Sullivan asserted that,

> A consensus has been reached, when the infant or child has learned the precisely right word for a situation, a word which means not only what it is thought to mean by the mothering one, but also means that to the infant (Sullivan, 1953).

Only then does a word have the "same" meaning for both. But, a word has meaning in this sense to the two persons only when it evokes similar responses or activities, which is its meaning. When a sign or a symbol evokes this sort of shared response or action, it has reached what Sullivan called the syntaxic mode of experience. Sullivan surmised that the first instances of syntaxic experience may occur between the twelfth and eighteenth month of the infant's extrauterine life.

Autistic language is an expression of what Sullivan called the parataxic mode of experience, which precedes the syntaxic mode of experience. In the parataxic mode there may be little consensus about what two or more people are talking about. One's experiences tend to be "associated" by the sequences or patterns of events in interpersonal relations, rather than grammatically or logically organized. Insufficient maturation and experience have not yet laid the groundwork for shared experiences, the use of language which has a common meaning and an orderly (grammatical) use of words, phrases, clauses and sentences. The latter requires several years of growth and is a gradual affair.

Reverie

Autistic language gradually merges with the great body of processes subsequently called *reverie*. At least to a degree, they are generically identical. At first, reverie processes, to some extent, are manifested by the baby's vocalizations in the absence of an audience. However, to some extent, reverie processes also occur in the presence of an audience. In reverie processes, the baby carries on a certain amount of exercise of his "language." Part of this is due to the apparent fact that he likes to listen to his own vocalizations and enjoys his increasing facility in the use of language. Up to and including the second year, whatever processes that go on are presumed to be purely autistic. Gradually, the child's overt use of language shifts from overt to silent speech. But after roughly his second year, his autistic reverie processes, when overt, will gradually evolve from audible to silent speech. Apart from cultural taboos, there is no good reason for this. But, the cultural taboos are very powerful and are communicated by the mother to her offspring. If her efforts in this connection do not suffice, when the youngster starts school, the ridicule of his peers will—although not always. Some children start school so badly warped that they are in grave need of psychiatric treatment of one sort or another.

Sullivan claimed that in later life, only those reverie processes which are in preparation for the expression of something, for the communication of something, may take on the attributes of the syntaxic mode. Otherwise, reverie continues to be more or less autistic, relatively untroubled by shared experience and grammatical rules. One should not forget that normal people carry on a great deal of *reverie*—that is pleasant musings or fantasies as in daydreams.

CHILDHOOD

In the lectures delivered during the last three or four years of his life, Sullivan seems to have more or less equated the autistic and the paratixic mode of experience. But, the more familiar "autistic" is more suited to communication in some contexts. Thus, if one says that much of the speech of a schizophrenic person is autistic (lacking in consensual validation), one is not likely to confuse a prospective clinician.

During infancy, the infant's ever-increasing ability to acquire language behavior very frequently is rewarded with "a very high premium" of tenderness. But, all through life, verbal behavior takes on truly marvelous attributes—not the least of which is to *confuse* thought.

It is interesting to note that the essence of magic may be characterized by a lack of any logical connection between means and ends in verbal behavior or overt actions.

There are times when Sullivan formulates his ideas with a force and skill that can hardly be duplicated. The following is an elegant illustration:

> The extraordinary value that comes to invest verbal behavior, especially as it manifests itself in the school years, is one of the important factors which make it difficult for us to be aware of reverie processes that are in a relatively simple parataxic mode of experience, or even of some reverie

processes that are in highly developed forms of the parataxic mode. Verbal behavior takes to itself, in the case of all those who are not born deaf-mutes, qualities bordering on the really magical; for instance, a good many of us, even though we are properly invested with the degree of doctor of this or that, show quite often and quite clearly that we depend on really magical potencies in certain of our verbal behaviors. And in psychiatric practice, we encounter chronological adults whose unearthly dependence on the potency of verbal behavior is, quite clearly, the outstanding characteristic of their difficulty with others (Sullivan, 1953).

LANGUAGE AND THE FUSION OF PERSONIFICATIONS

In the early part of childhood, largely because of the peculiar power of language, there is a *fusion of personifications insofar as consciousness is concerned.* The mother has one name "Mama," which she calls herself; and perhaps some others, relatives, neighbors, when they talk to the child do so as well. This of course goes hand in hand with the increasing maturation of the child. Nevertheless, the dichotomy of Good and Bad Mother may continue at lower levels of awareness. The fusion of the two may not be complete. Thus, in later life, there is evidence that, under certain circumstances, the person may seek someone who will fairly closely fit the personification of the good mother—or aspects of the mothering one which the real mother never had. Thanks to the power of language, and to the unique power that is put on the acquisition of language, the personifications of one stage of development enter into personifications at a later stage, though this very seldom occurs totally.

THE THEOREM OF ESCAPE

Those who genuinely love children (in contrast to some parental figures who regard them as extensions of themselves) may sometimes observe certain very sad occurrences when a group of youngsters are engaged in play. It may happen that one child acts so aggressively that he is soon ignored or ostracized by the others. Or, on another occasion, one may observe a child standing on the periphery of his world—his playmates who are busy with some game—silent, inactive, wistful, alone. He knows he is not accepted or approved. Since there is no evidence that children are born with any given tendency toward this or that pattern of interpersonal relations, one can assume that the parents have already unwittingly accomplished a good deal of evil in their upbringing of the soon-to-be isolated child.

In other words, during the first five or six years of life, the self-system of the growing child normally acquires a particular organization, whose quality, character, and direction have been shaped by the parents. The self-system is extraordinarily resistant to change by experience. So, by reason of its organization and functional activity, it tends to escape influence by experience which is inconsistent with its current organization and fuctional activity operating in a communal environment. Although the self develops stage by stage, it tends to adhere to the organization which was built at the start; it acts like blinders. One may clearly perceive what is in one's field of perception and cognition, but, under normal circumstances, not a great deal more. Outside this field of awareness lies the vast unknown. If one could step outside the margin of the self, one does not know what anxieties might threaten him. Moreover, it is the self which organizes one's experience and provides life with meaning and comparative safety.

But, the limiting restrictive power of the self is not absolute. Sullivan asserts that all additions to or modifications of the self-system are either *imperfect observations* of the circumstances that have caused anxiety, and of the successful interventions of the self-system to minimize or avoid repetition of these circumstances, or certain *definite interventions by which more complex operations are built out of simpler ones, that is new things are made out of the old.* Perhaps this is the essence of a good deal of creativity. Moreover, culture is said to be based on no single great general principle that can be grasped and assimilated by a genius, but is based instead on many contradictory principles (1953). At this point, it is well to recall that it was due to education for the life in our culture that we have all experienced a great deal of anxiety.

Ordinarily, we do not become anxious in connection with the satisfaction of somatic needs. Thus, the manifestations of any dynamism in the satisfaction of needs may be enhanced and modified by recurrent experience. Our self-esteem may be enhanced by the belief that we are becoming sophisticated with regard to the exposure to the pleasures of life.

It is the manifestations of any dynamism in the fulfillment of various cultural demands and performances with which we are not accustomed that may cause trouble. Frequently, they require patterns of interpersonal relations which are foreign to the self. A single brief excursion in a culture not too radically different from his own may, if one is secure and self-confident, be exciting rather than threatening, but let one venture into a totally different culture — say, an anthropology student — he may be unable to withstand the implicit challenge to his own *Weltanschauung* (world view). That is chiefly the reason that newcomers to the United States from various foreign countries have tended to cluster in cultural ghettoes until they become more or less "assimilated"—if they ever do.

Every human society has a complex network of interpersonal relations. If the foreigner is a tourist visiting, he will generally be tolerated—within limits. Hence, the tourist does not usually suffer loss of self-esteem, at least during a brief stay. But if a visitor to a foreign country plans a prolonged stay, he will have to learn the customs of the country as best he can, their patterns of interpersonal relations and, however imperfectly, their language. Otherwise, he will endure recurrent experiences that may entail a whole series of failures in his attempts at security operations and successful adjustment. The reason is that his self-respect is at stake. In fact, if the foreigner does not acquire a working knowledge of the culture patterns of the new country, he will not be able to relate to others or survive in their society.

Unfortunately, essentially similar problems face us at home, in the country in which we live. We never come in contact with, let alone assimilate, the entire culture of our society. If our parents are educationally restricted or psychologically warped, we are likely to be at a considerable disadvantage. Even in a familiar milieu, urban life chronically presents us with unfamiliar or unusual patterns of interpersonal relations. To the degree that the self-esteem has been damaged, one can go through a whole series of consistent failures of security operations without learning much, if he learns anything at all, in his attempts to relate to others. Perhaps the greatest enemy of personal change is selective inattention. The more insecure one is, the more frequently one is likely to employ it in situations where he might otherwise profit from experience. If a person becomes badly warped in the course of development, he will very likely require prolonged treatment before he can overcome the more severe limitations he has acquired.

SUBLIMATION

Sullivan believed that a great deal of what is called learning—chiefly education in interpersonal relations, whether real or imaginary or a "blend" of both—is due to what he called his variant of *sublimation*. In rudimentary form, it appears first in late infancy, becomes conspicuous in childhood, and in the succeeding eras becomes remarkably prominent. In classical Freudian theory, sublimation pertains chiefly to sexuality and aggression. Not so in Sullivan's theory.

> Sublimation is the unwitting substitution, for a behavior pattern which encounters anxiety or collides with the self-esteem, of a socially more acceptable activity pattern which satisfies part of the motivational system that caused trouble (Sullivan, 1953).

Sullivan claimed that by unwitting or unnoted, he was referring to the "great congeries" or aggregation of covert referential processes which must have occurred, but whose occurrence is completely unknown to the person concerned. These processes can only be inferred from what the individual does know and does notice, and how he acts. The classical example of how one proceeds from the known to the unknown is dream interpretation. Symbol processes occurring in sleep —dreams— provide an outlet for the rest of the unsatisfied need in more fortunate circumstances. Apart from somatic needs, it is theoretically possible for any cultural (acquired) need to be sublimated if it becomes invested with anxiety. Except in the case of those who have been badly warped, sublimation is not only a benign but an essential process. Life is much too short to provide a rational explanation if one wishes, to teach a child why things have to be learned. In a perfectly rational culture this might not be necessary. Failure to understand this can cause teachers in the primary grades, school psychologists, and counselors of all sorts to injure rather than help some of their more insecure charges.

The disintegration of the dynamisms of personality under a totally coercive social environment, as in Totalitarian Societies (brain washing), is, of course, not to be compared with the disintegration of behavior patterns which may occur during individual child rearing as a result of anxiety. The disintegration of personality structure need not end with childhood as the common occurrences of psychotic disintegration of chronological adolescents and adults seem to indicate.

The disintegration of behavior patterns begins in childhood. Sullivan claimed this chiefly occurs in family groups that are not estimable in the skill, ingenuity, and understanding with which they try to discharge their social responsibilities.

Thus, the first instances of the disintegration of behavior patterns and of patterns of covert processes, he thought, took place under the force of anxiety quite early in childhood. These disintegrations may get "somewhere near" the area of the "not-me" personification. They are no longer part of the growing self-structure. However, one has to consider the character of the need which remains as part of the self and, as such, continues to exert its influence. When the need is retained, a large part of living becomes rather disorganized, because more and more anxiety piles up in the face of the mothering one's disapproval. In the former instance, when the patterns of behavior and covert processes are disintegrated, they do not become sublimated, but recombine in complex patterns of activities, a number of which may develop into mental disorder, as in the case of malevolence. Another possibility when patterns of behavior and covert processes have to be disintegrated is *regression* or a reactivation of earlier patterns.

THE THEOREM OF RECIPROCAL EMOTION

How many thousands of times has one — sadly — observed two people involved or "integrated" in a situation working at cross purposes? Each may engage in self-defeating purposes. Sullivan formulated a general statement which applies not only to such self-defeating behavior but to the fostering and enhancing of interpersonal relations as well. The implications of the "theorem" are very broad. It is formulated as follows:

> Integration in an interpersonal situation is a reciprocal process in which (1) complementary needs are resolved, or aggravated; (2) reciprocal patterns of activity are developed, or disintegrated; and (3) foresight of satisfaction, or rebuff of similar needs is facilitated (Sullivan, 1953).

The paradigm which Sullivan employs is that of mother and child. Normally, the mother has a need to act tenderly and the child has a need to receive tenderness. But a mother who may be unable to fulfill this need may "cause" the child's need to be aggravated. Tenderness is conveyed in numerous ways, but should never be confused with "smother love." The atttitude of tenderness is communicated by numerous patterns of activity, ranging from smiles, tones of voice, an alertness to the child's vulnerability, and to encouragements of his growing abilities and skills. The child increasingly develops joyful activities and learns how to rely on mother for guidance in the enhancement of various skills; to seek help in his exploratory activities. In so far as the mother encourages and assists the child's efforts by numerous tender attitudes and overt behaviors, the child will tend to anticipate more and more such delights, and possibly others he has observed, in the future.

The inadequate mother will tend to look upon the child's simply wondrous activities as a nuisance or worse. Hence, his efforts become frustrated and dulled. In this instance (2) as in (1), he encounters so much anxiety that many of his activities are disintegrated. Thus, when the mother is inadequate, her child starts out from very early in life with an increasing desire for various needs such as tenderness. If he is not loved, a beginning conviction occurs that he is inadequate and inferior because he does not measure up to his mother's demands or the skills he observes that other children are developing, and a foreboding that various of his needs and lost activities promise nothing for the future but misery. To extend the illustration, once he starts school, the child's failures are likely to be exaggerated. And this may continue indefinitely. In extreme cases, he may become malevolent. Needless to say, there may be shades and gradations of inadequacy in a child who has suffered such unfortunate experience. Barring extraordinary good fortune in school, the negative side of this process can continue indefinitely. But, all too often, even in school, the efforts of an acute school psychologist may be thwarted by the parents. Their child, they say, was always good and they will tolerate no meddling by strangers. Or they will flatly deny that the teacher is telling the truth. People will often try to preserve their self-esteem at great cost to themselves, and sometimes to others.

MAL-DEVELOPMENTS IN THE SELF-SYSTEM

Sullivan claimed that, with the increase of pressure toward socialization of the young, the *negative side* of the *reciprocal process* of emotional patterns tends to be accentuated; that needs are aggravated because they are thwarted; and that patterns of activity have to be sublimated or disintegrated. Further, in certain cases, as was previously mentioned, rebuff is anticipated of a large part of one's future living. These situations tend to fit into the self called "bad-me."

In childhood, children may begin to learn propitiatory gestures and verbal patterns. For example, in the first or second grade, some of them learn to be remarkably "sweet" and well-behaved in class, but once they escape the teacher's eye this can change. But, the particular propitiatory gesture we are concerned with has to do with verbal behavior. The parents teach the child that when he is bad — perhaps he has repeated some unmentionable word he has picked up — mother may say, "That is a disgusting word. Say you're sorry or I will slap you." And the child who is no fool, sooner or later learns that when he says, "I'm sorry, Ma" it has a remarkable effect. For some mysterious reason, mother's anger is assuaged. This is a very simple illustration of how the child learns propitiatory verbal behavior. And this "magic" may persist through life.

Imagine a college student who dates a female classmate. For one reason or another, he treats her abominally with the result that as far as she is concerned he is thenceforth worse than poison. However, the boy has not yet learned that the young lady whom he dated comes from a conservative home and is not, "easy." Soon after, when he telephones her and is met with icy disdain he tries to tell her how sorry he is, that he meant on harm, and, furthermore, certain teachers have declared outright in class or have implied that sexual relations are "healthy." A young man or woman, because of his or her "medieval" moral code, runs the risk of becoming "neurotic." Nevertheless, our imaginary young lady expresses contempt toward casual sexual behavior. Our imaginary young man is puzzled if not chagrined. Has he not said he was very sorry and regretted his behavior? Why do not these apologies (verbal stratagems) wash away the hurt, angry feelings of the "puritanical" girl? One could use numerous examples from every day life. The point, of course, is not to belittle courtesy whose essence someone — it may have been Oscar Wilde — said is respect for the other fellow's feelings. Nevertheless, during childhood and the next (juvenile) era, youngsters learn that various combinations of words when skillfully employed sometimes have a truly magical effect. ("Say you are sorry".) Unfortunately there are people who rely on magical verbal statements when there is no hope it will succeed — quite the contrary. An extreme example is the person who suffers an obsessive-compulsive neurosis.

During childhood, something striking is said to happen to one of the components of the generic need for tenderness which characterizes infants while they are still very young: the need for *physical contact*. For reasons that Sullivan does not make very clear, there is an elaboration of this need, first as a need for participants and later as a need for an audience. Of course, during infancy normally there is a good deal of tenderness by the mothering one expressed through physical contact. Many recent investigators have emphasized the importance of touching as a modality of transaction between mother and infant. Touching is thought to be extremely important, especially for primative babies who are particularly difficult babies to relate to (Brazelton, 1975).

At any rate, Sullivan adds that late infants and young children like most emphatically to play with mother, to engage in certain exercises with mother which satisfy certain zonal muscular needs, as in manual activity, and so on. At a still later stage they have a definite preference, he says, for putting on their performances in the presence of the tenderness-giving, approval-giving elders.

However, sometimes owing to various circumstances, such as unavailability of the mothering one, because of too many other children in the home, too many demands of other kinds on the mother, mental disorder on her part, or ("crazy" ideas she has about the child's will), the child meets with such consistent rebuff of his expressed needs for tenderness that his overt behavior and covert processes are thwarted. The rebuff of the need for tenderness results in the change of the child's behavior regarding his expression of this need. In some instances, the youngster is able to sublimate his behavior and he regains tenderness from his mother because, it may be, he makes fewer demands and becomes more "helpful" around the house. But, a good many children do not regain tenderness despite their efforts and are compelled to disintegrate the behavior patterns and covert processes, which in happier circumstances would be manifested as the need for tenderness, because, quite realistically, they foresee rebuff of any overt expression of this need. The experience of such children and young juveniles may vary from a slap in the face to an eloquently disdainful expression on mother's face. Then the child or juvenile becomes "mischievous." And mischievous behavior can cover a wide range and can grow to a point where mother in later years may be made to suffer dearly, although she may or may not know what started it. For example, the parents may be quite conscious of the fact that they were much more tender toward the *last* child in a series of offspring. Thus, an uninformed observer may wonder why the child is much more friendly than his brothers and sisters.

MALEVOLENCE, HATRED AND ISOLATING TECHNIQUES

In childhood, a new educative influencce is brought to bear on the child, namely, fear, frequently associated with anxiety. It is a new educative influence, since it is a fear of the parent's or parent surrogates to impose pain often combined with anxiety. Sullivan pointed out many times that when one experiences fear, the circumstances provoking it can frequently be analyzed, identified, and assimilated in foresight for the future. In the case of relatively *mild anxiety* that is only relatively true at best. During childhood, when the parents are attempting to educate their offspring according to their lights, he almost always begins to learn certain indices or cues which enable him to catch on to the situations when it is extremely unsafe to violate authority, and also those situations where he has a chance to escape punishment. Normally, the child begins to discriminate father from mother, that is, two different authority figures. This proves useful, because it is the source of information that will be reasonably dependable in foreseeing the course of events, which is, of course, a vital clue to what future interpersonal relations, at least in certain respects, will be like.

Such reflections lead directly to Sullivan's notion which follows: Insofar, he said,

> as the authority figures are confusing to the child and insofar as the authority situations are incongruous from time to time so that, according to the measure of the child's maturing abilities and experiences, there is no making sense of them—then, even before the end of the thirtieth month, let us say, we see instances in which the child is already beginning to suffer a deterioration of development of high-grade foresight (Sullivan, 1953).

For some reasons, Sullivan thought it quite probable for those who suffer such misfortune in later stages of development that conscious exercise of foresight, witting study of how to get to a more or less recognized goal, will not be very highly developed.

The formal training of the child includes "imposing the prescriptions of the culture on the child." These prescriptions are said to be often most glaringly contradictory on different occasions, so that they require a complex discrimination of authority situations. For many years, children will not be able to comprehend the possible reasonableness of cultural prescriptions — if ever. (These ideas were promulgated a generation ago. At the present time it is becoming increasingly unclear in our culture as to what prescriptions most parents under 30 teach their children.)

A great many children learn, or have learned, to conceal and deceive the parents mainly because of the "irrational and impulse driven type of education by anxiety" and by reward and punishment (tenderness and fear) to which they have been subjected (1953). These children develop the ability to conceal what is going on in them from the authority figures and, thus, deceive them. Sullivan, who was by no means a sentimentalist, said some of the ability children develop to conceal and deceive is "literally" taught by the authoritative figures. And some of it is acquired by trial and error learning from human example. One is tempted to wonder what would happen to them if the children, by some miracle, in the United States learned to be always truthful and good. Would they be a spectacular success in business? Or in their professions?

In any case, the growing abilities of a great many children to conceal and to deceive gradually tend to evolve into verbalisms or rationalizations and *as if* performances. There does not seem to be any necessity to dwell on verbalisms, except to mention at this point that, to a remarkable degree, they constitute elements of functional mental disorder. Although rationalizations are designed to evade anxiety, they become a function of the self-system's tendency to escape from (potentially educative) experience not congruent with its current directions.

As if performances are divided into two divisions, one of which is an absolutely inevitable part of everyone's maturing through childhood, namely *dramatizations*. In regard to dramatizations, by means of a species of play-acting, a child first learns to *act like* the mothering one and *sound* like her also. As the father becomes more conspicuous around the house, he too becomes a model, although normally the male child more or less abandons his play acting of imitating mother by the time he reaches the juvenile era, while the female child is rapidly learning how to be feminine. Of course, this dichotomy never gets to be absolute. From acting like the parent, the child probably progresses along these *as if* performances to trying to *act as if one were* the authority figure.

It may happen that a child retains or acquires so many attributes of the parent of the other sex that he (or she) never achieves complete masculinity or femininity as the case may be, in accordance with cultural definitions. For example, a mother who dearly wants a girl may find that nature has presented her with a boy. She may then proceed to rear him as if he were a girl and do her best to isolate him from the male roughnecks he encounters. There are many possibilities, including situations where a submissive father abandons his attempts to teach his son to act like a boy. Furthermore, in the eyes of the child, the father may seem to be an unworthy model. On the other hand, mother may be rather aggressive but more worthy in the child's eyes.

Over the last generation, the field of normal and abnormal human sexuality has been considerably elucidated. Stoller's (1968) concept of "core gender identity," which is the conviction established in the first two or three years of life that one belongs to the male or to the female sex is very close to what Sullivan (1953) called "gender lines."

It is thought today that core-gender identity is created by multiple factors such as: biological (embryological and central nervous system centers) and genital anatomy (which serves as a signal for parents that they have a boy or a girl). Sex assignment and rearing (parents personalities and attitudes about the offspring's maleness and masculinity, or femaleness and feminity), classical visceral and operant conditioning (the effect of being raised from birth by female or male), and possibly imprinting (which is known in some birds and mammals) Stoller (1953). Sullivan concentrated mainly on the interperosnal aspect of the "gender lines" and stressed that the additions to the personified self on the specific basis of whether one is a boy or a girl are advanced notably by two influences: (1) The child's play at being the authority of his own sex; and (2) rewards and punishments, interest and approval, and the influence of shame and guilt (Sullivan, 1953).

The other group of performances is called *preoccupations*. Preoccupation as a way of dealing with fear-provoking situations or the threat of punishment, and of avoiding or minimizing anxiety is said to appear quite early in life. The child learns that preoccupation with some particular *one time* interesting and probably profitable activity is very valuable to continue because it tends to ward off punishment and anxiety imposed by irrational authority. Should it come about that such performances of the child are not only successful in avoiding punishment and anxiety but also provoke tenderness and approval, he is starting on a course that will be strikingly complex and *obsessional*.

The final topic which forms the background toward the development of malevolence is *anger* and the peculiar form it takes is resentment. Certain children who have not previously experienced physical restraint manifest rage. Although not previously mentioned, it should be said that Sullivan believed physical restraint "calls out" rage even in infants, often observed as temper tantrums. When a young child of 30 months is undergoing physical punishment which entails some physical restraint, he suffers fear leading to rage, "a symbolic discharge of a high degree of anger." But *rage behavior* has no efficacy or value in such situations (Sullivan, 1956). And so what might be called a version of its felt component, anger, becomes quite important. In certain circumstances, children learn that anger, in various settings and accompanied by various behavioral trappings does work, either with other children, or the authority figures, or both. For example, mother may become upset because her child, for some evident or unknown reason, is angry. So, the youngster may arouse a lot of attention from mother and possibly a dish of those delicious cherries in the refrigerator which were promised as dessert. Of course, in some homes children are "well trained" in the use of anger, and in certain unhappy homes children well into the school years have *tantrums*, which are essentially unmodified rage behavior, because anger does not work. Thus, one occasionally observes a child who literally perpetrates a tantrum on the sidewalk with a great deal of yelling and thrashing about until the harried mother drops the groceries and rallies round. And this, of course, tends to reinforce the youngster's tendency toward rage behavior. Such a tendency does not bode well for his future development.

In more typical homes, it may happen that the child discovers, perhaps quite by accident, that anger is sometimes a potent instrument for warding off anxiety. Anger is often less painful than anxiety; and one does not usually feel quite so helpless. This stratagem is also often unwittingly employed by adults.

Sullivan asserted that, in a great many other unfortunate homes, children develop a complex modification of anger, that is, resentment in order to ward off punishment. The child may be occupied with some task or activity which, as far as he knows is "perfectly all right." Yet for some, to him, inexplicable reason he is suddenly punished and made anxious because of the mysteriously forbidden activity. However, he may be punished for an activity for which he knows he will be punished, but it is so attractive he refuses to abandon it. In such circumstances, a great many children resort to resentment instead of anger which would only aggravate the situation. Anger becomes circumvented by *resentment*, which is modified anger and has very important cover aspects. In the "most awkward type of home situation" these covert processes are said to be complciated by efforts to conceal even the resentment, because it might bring further punishment. If this kind of situation, at almost any stage of life, becomes chronic, the tensions which cannot be allowed direct expression may be "diverted" into the gastrointestinal tract. One's spouse, for example, may, for one reason or another, including the character of her self-system, be compelled to conceal her resentment at significnt others and may one day "come up" with a gastric or duodenal ulcer.

It should be quite clear that Sullivan believed that no one is born with evil propensities. Unfortunately, there is so much evil in the world, very frequently due to complex political, economic, or religious conditions that the notion of a *destructive instinct* is very appealing to some people. Although "participant observers" have questionable competence in explaining the conditions which give rise to various political, economic, or religious conflicts, some of them—including Freud and Sullivan—have fancied that they have some peculiar formula to explain the causes or cures of those usually disastrous states of affairs. Sullivan believed that psychiatric insights, if wisely applied, could alleviate the tensions that cause wars. It is true, however, that in many past or present conflicts, the mental states of the participants have exacerbated those ghastly wars.

In the understanding of "two groups" (a transaction of two people) and groups of larger but still small size as in group psychotherapy, Sillivan has a lot to offer. Hence, we can learn a great deal from what he has to say about *malevolence*. Since a rose smells just as sweet by any other name, one may say that some people learn to be evil, though they were not born with destructive tendencies.

Sullivan flatly declared that, because of their experience, some children become *malevolent*, although he seems originally to have thought it "shows" first during the juvenile era. Malevolencce has several manifestations. Sullivan claimed that there are so-called timid children whose malevolence is manifested by their being so afraid to do anything that they just always fail to do things that are most urgently desired. But, the outstanding and notoriously great group are those who are frankly mischievous and then evolve to be the type of person, the potential bully, who "takes it out" on some younger member of the family, or a neighbor's child, pets, and so on, indefinitely. Since Sullivan gave these lectures a generation ago, malevolence in various forms seems much more widespread.

For a variety of reasons, many children are said to have the experience that when they need tenderness, when they do the things which once brought tender cooperation from mother, they are not only denied tenderness but they are treated in a fashion that arouses anxiety, or in some instances, even pain. Normally, children are wonderful people and there are still many persons who delight in caring for them and watching them grow—in contrast to those who regard them as a burden, who restrict their freedom, and who destroy those wonderful exciting early days. The reader, whose contact with children may be very limited indeed in these days of small American families, must try to realize that today's children are in many ways as different from himself as are his grandparents. Although children are by no means as helpless as infants, they are still terribly vulnerable vis-à-vis parents who have little time to devote to them, or are indifferent or even hostile or cruel. Among working class mothers, the hostility or cruelty may be frequently manifested in the street or in the supermarket where children love to survey the cornucopia of delicious foods. Middle class mothers, who are better educated and more sophisticated, may be much more circumspect in their manifestations of hostility or cruelty. For example, it is a simple matter to lock the child in his room when he is "bad" or to prevent him for considerable periods of time from playing with other children because he is "sick." But, mother has much more subtle ways of venting her hostility or cruelty on the child and these are the most destructive of all.

It may come about that he may discover that when he manifests the need for tenderness toward the parent figures around him, he frequently is disadvantaged, made anxious, or made fun of, with the result that he feels hurt or in some cases literally hurt by, for example, a solid slap across the face. Yet so powerful is the need for tenderness that he may seek it again and again — with invariably the same results. Finally, it is borne in upon him — and he eventually becomes quite clear about it — that it is highly disadvantageous to manifest any need for tender cooperation from the authoritative figure around him. He learns that it will only bring him anxiety or pain. Consequently, when he feels a need for tender cooperation, he "shows" something else — and this is the conviction that he lives among enemies, an idea which may forever appear in his attitudes toward persons, especially authoritative figures in various walks of life. Hence, the development of malevolence can easily flower into a vicious reciprocal process. One of the worst outcomes of malevolence is that, in the next era, when it tends to become solidified, the youngster becomes convinced that he really is no good. Is he not surrounded by others who seem to be treated with kindness and respect? Hence, it is logical for him to wonder: What is so wrong with me? And when he arrives in the first or second grade, the teacher who may have studied all the right courses in college, unless she is a very secure individual, may quickly find herself baffled and confused by this child who may have learned a plethora of mischievous techniques.

Unless the child's experience has been so crippling that he is unable to learn very much, his self-system is still developing. But, almost inevitably, he will have a "negative self-image." Or, in Sullivan's language, the personified self is prevailingly "bad-me." Of course, it may happen that he unwittingly tries to dissociate so much of his behavior that "not-me" has been growing also. The teachers are mistreating him for one reason or another. Why, parents may tell you, when he is home he acts as though he were virtually an angel.

The malevolent transformation needs to be emphasized. The child's mischievous behavior may evolve into the malevolent transformation if it is not already a symptom of it. He may become a juvenile delinquent or, subsequently, turn to a life of crime.

REFERENCES

Allport, G. *Pattern and Growth in Personality*. Holt, Rinehart and Winston, New York, 1961.

American Psychiatric Association, Task Force on Nomenclature and Statistics. *DSM III —Diagnostic and Statistical Manual of Mental Disorders* 3rd ed., Washington, D.C., APA, 1980.

Brazelton, T.B. Mother infant neonatal separation: Some delayed consequences, in Leiderman, P.H. and Seashore, M.J., *Parents Infants Interaction*. Ciba Foundation Symposium 33 Associated Scientific Publishers, New York, 1975.

Ferguson, C.A. Baby talk in six languages, in Gumperz, M.J., Hymes, D., and Menasha, eds., *The Ethography of Communication*. Am. Anthropologist. Special publication of the American Anthropological Association, 1964–1966.

Slobin, D. On the nature of talk to children, in Lenneberg, E. and Lenneberg, E., eds., *Foundations of Language Development I*. Academic Press, New York, 1975.

Snow, C. Mother's speech to children learning language. *Child Dev. 1972; 43: 549–564*.

Stern, D. *The First Relationship*. Harvard University Press, Cambridge, 1977.

Stoller, R.J. Gender identity, in Freedman, A.M., Kaplan, H.L., and Sadak, B.S., *Comprehensive Textbook of Psychiatary II*. Williams and Wilkins, Baltimore, 1980.

Stoller, R.J. *Sex and Gender*. Science House, New York, 1968.

Sullivan, H.S. *The Interpersonal Theory of Psychiatry*. W.W. Norton, New York, 1953.

Sullivan, H.S. *Clinical Studies in Psychiatry*. W.W. Norton, New York, 1956.

4

The Transition from Childhood

THE MEANING OF ARREST OF DEVELOPMENT

In the first chapter, Freud's notion of *fixation* and Sullivan's notion of an *arrest of development* were used rather loosely, as if they were synonymous. But, they are not. Freud formulated fixation as a partial or more or less total halt of libidinal development. For him the paradigm of fixation is sexual. Of course, other psychoanalysts who claim to belong to the Freudian school may broaden or modify this and other Freudian concepts. It is rare these days to find a masterly and undiluted explication of the essentials of Freud's psychology such as Brenner's. In any case, Sullivan stated that arrest of development does *not* imply that things have become static, and that, henceforth, the person will remain just as he was in any essential aspect as he was at the time that development was arrested. He further asserted that the conspicuous evidence of arrest and deviation of development is, at first, a delay in the "showing" of change which characterizes the statistically usual course, and later, the appearance of eccentricities of interpersonal relations. Although by no means self-evident, they are signs of the developmental experiences which have been missed or sadly distorted. But, the freedom and velocity of constructive change are said to be very markedly reduced.

A Sullivanian psycotherapist always seeks out the *specific* arrests of development his patient suffered. This discovery often provides additional important clues as to "what ails the patient," because such arrests of development have, so to speak, helped make the patient what he is when he seeks professional help, and their understanding may make his current difficulties more intelligible.

GENDER AS A FACTOR IN THE PERSONIFICATION OF THE SELF

All too often, gender is confused with sex. Sex is essentially a biological attribute. Gender is basically a psychological trait. Not surprisingly, the two are interrelated as, in general, the biological and psychological features of man are. According to Sullivan and others, sexuality forms a continuum.

To a large degree, masculinity and femininity are acquired. Sullivan claimed that the child is influenced psychologically by the fact that the parent who is of the same sex as the child has a feeling of familiarity with him (or her), while the parent of the opposite sex has a surviving feeling of difference and of uncertainty. This phenomenon may or may not be subtly woven into the parents' behavior, so that for some years it may remain selectively inattended. Sullivan thought that the father feels more comfortable with his sons, than with his daughters. So, the father believes that he is right in his expectations of his sons. Be that as it may, a normal father will leave the upbringing of his daughters to his wife, who additionally becomes a model of femininity at least for several years, a fact of which Sullivan was well aware. *Pari-passu*, the same applies to the father in relation to his sons. Doubtless, a cultural factor enters into this matter. In an agricultural society, for example, the father is likely to prefer six strong sons to six strong daughters.

There are other considerations regarding gender as a factor in the personification of self. There is for example the child's play at being the authority figure of his own sex. A boy who plays the expected roles of the authority figure, if the latter is the father, gets rewarded. Otherwise, the boy is treated with indifference and disapproval. The girl's situation is analogous.

Sullivan may or may not be right in thinking that this gender preference had "something to do" with Freud's formulation of the Oedipus complex. Early in his career, some of Freud's patients, who were female hysterics, repeatedly recounted stories of how when they were children, an older man, such as an uncle or a father, had seduced them or at least made sexual overtures. For a time, Freud believed these fancies, until at length he "recognized" them for what he thought they were: long-repressed sexual attractions toward their fathers or father surrogates. Then, he became convinced that little boys had similar wishes regarding their mothers. Some have speculated that Freud's relationship to his own mother, whose outstanding favorite he was, may have also influenced him, but it is not profitable to pursue this line of speculation. It is also true that Freud thought that parents tend to favor members of the opposite sex, for reasons that have a sexual tinge, but we shall not pursue this idea either.

Regardless of Sullivan's interpretation of the Oedipus complex, he did have valuable ideas about the development of femininity and masculinity, which have been previously touched upon. He stated that the additions to the personified self ("I" or "Me") on the specific basis of whether one is a boy or a girl are advanced notably by two influences. The child's play at being the authority figure—as in the case where children in play act out different roles—is one influence. The second is the influence which can also be observed chiefly with regard to rewards and punishments, especially interest and approval in contrast with indifferences and disapproval exerted by the parents or their surrogates. Sullivan said that these influences tend to educate the child with peculiar facility in the social expectations of his particular sex (gender), and to inculcate many of the cultural prescriptions. For example, when the female child learns, chiefly by trial and error from human example, something that seems very feminine, she gets applause, interest, and support from the mother—depending, of course upon the mother's view of femininity. An analogous situation occurs with the boy and his father.

SCHECTER'S INTERPRETATION OF THE OEDIPUS COMPLEX VERSUS SULLIVAN AND OTHERS

An interpretation of the Oedipus complex from a quasi-interpersonal point of view by the psychoanalyst David E. Schecter provides a perspective that differs considerably from both Freud and Sullivan. In a paper titled "The Oedipus Complex: Considerations of Ego Development and Parental Interaction," Schecter (1968) examines two aspects in the emergence and resolution "of the Oedipal phase of human development." These two aspects are

> (1) the contribution of the child's ego (cognitive-affective) development; and
> (2) the nature of the parental and family response and its transactional or "feed-back" influence on this development.

Apparently, Schecter had difficulty attempting to define the term Oedipus Complex. He quotes, with approval, Erikson's attempt to define "Oedipus Complex" as the latter stated it in *Childhood and Society* (1950). Erikson's statement runs as follows:

> This term, of course, has complicated matters in that it compares what is to be inferred from a story of King Oedipus. The name thus establishes an analogy between two unknowns. The idea is that Oedipus, who inadvertently killed his father and married his mother, become a mythical hero and on the stage is viewed with intense pity and terror because to possess one's mother is a universal wish, universally tabooed.

Psychoanalysis verifies in daily work the simple conclusion that boys attach their first genital affection to the maternal adults who have otherwise given affection to their bodies and develop their first sexual rivalry against the genital owners of those maternal persons. To conclude, as Diderot did, that if the little boy had the power of a man, he would rape his mother and murder his father is meaningless. For if he had such power he would not be a child and would not need to stay with his parents — in which case he might simply prefer other sex objects. As it is, infantile genitality attaches itself to the protectors and ideals of childhood and suffers internal complications therefrom (Schecter, 1968).

Schecter mentions a paper published by Freud in 1931 on "Female Sexuality" which showed that he had become deeply impressed with the impact of pre-Oedipal experience on the development of the Oedipal phase. Certain statements in Freud's paper led to an intensified study by psychoanalysts, in order to discover the earlier developments in the child's relation to his parents. Schecter (1968) notes two important omissions in this search which suggested two important lines of development in psychoanalytic theory:

1. The child had been discussed without much regard to the structural aspect of his ego at any given stage of its development. This lack gave rise to an intensified study of ego psychology, especially in a developmental framework.

2. The child had been considered to develop according to a rather fixed instinctual "ground-plan" (oral, anal, phallic); little regard had been given to the specific family and cultural milieu that constitute varied and powerful forces shaping the young ego.

Schecter asserts that from this need developed the "cultural schools" which, however, have rarely operated with a detailed framework ("structure") of ego development. (With regard to Sullivan, this statement is partially inaccurate, since Sullivan's ideas about the self were influenced by William James and others who preceded Freud.) While the origins of interpersonal psychiatry were dealt with in *Psychoanalysis and Interpersonal Psychiatry* (Mullahy, 1970) at some length, it is important to mention that Sullivan developed his "theory" of interpersonal psychiatry chiefly from his study of schizophrenics, although to a certain extent he ultimately followed Freud's ground plan. Freud rarely worked with schizophrenics and had no theoretical framework to guide Sullivan in his work with them. (This is not to say he did not utilize certain insights of Freud including his dynamic orientation.) After a brief discussion of research in pre-Oedipal Ego Development, Schecter (1968) writes:

In brief, whereas originally the social attachment to mother was seen to be based on the relief of biological needs (hunger, cold, and so forth), including the need for oral gratification and later, contact needs, more recently the role of distance receptor stimulation is seen as a powerful source of the social attachment. To go a step further, we would emphasize that *mutual stimulation and responsiveness* —for example, mutual visual regard, smiling, vocalization, touch, imitation, games and communication—become the fabric of the infant's first social relationship and the mother-child bond.

Schecter's framework of ego development in children is not systematic. However, it does complement and tends to verify empirically some of Sullivan's ideas on infancy and childhood, as well as the recent experimental and observational research work that we referred to previously (see Stern, 1977).

It does not seem that Freud's meaning of the Oedipus Complex is as obscure as Schecter and others would have it. Even though Schecter points out that Freud modified his formulation during the course of his professional life, it seems that he was reasonably clear about what he meant when he wrote *An Outline of Psychoanalysis* (Freud, 1949).

> The boy enters the Oedipus phase; he begins to manipulate his penis, and simultaneously has phantasies of carrying out some sort of activity with it in relation to his mother; but at last, owing to the combined effect of a *threat of castration* and the spectacle of women's lack of a penis, he experiences the greatest trauma of his life . . .

It is perfectly clear that a boy, roughly ranging from age three to five—so Freud believed—has sexual fantasies about his mother, wants to kiss her, caress her, watch her undress, sleep with her at night, and so manipulates his penis and simultaneously has fantasies of carrying out some sort of activity with it in relation to his mother. But, the castration dread intervenes and forces the little boy to repress his incestuous wishes. While it seems clear that a boy of three, four, or five (leaving aside questions of maturation and learning) does not know the mechanisms of sexual intercourse, Freud leaves no doubt that for the little boy, his penis is the sexual organ around which, so to speak, his sexual wishes revolve. Schecter does not adequatley recognize this. And in effect he tells why. Schecter (1968) wrote:

> It is probably fair to say that the family structure creates the Oedipal situation; however, it is equally true that the infant's biological helplessness seems to have demanded some form of family caretaking arrangement.

This is a far cry from Freud's idea that the Oedipus Complex as he formulated it is universal and biologically ordained.

But, we must not "throw out the baby with the Oedipal bath." The essence of Schecter's paper has to do with ego development and parental transaction. In the first year of life, there is a progression, from behavior that can at the beginning be described mainly in physiologic terms, to behavior that comes to be endowed with "psychologic" and symbolic significance. A discrimination of self from non-self, and discrimination of mother as a very special being occurs. In addition, Schecter asserts, there are "the beginnings of internal mental representation of each of these categories of experience." Observation reveals the infant's increasingly selective and preferential smiling, vocalizing, visual, and receptive behaviors in relation to mother and as against other persons. Two dramatic forms of behavior may appear at around seven to eight months, revealing the intense specific attachment to mother. Even in her presence, a *reaction to strangers*, ranging from mild, sobering, staring expression may appear, an expression with inhibition, aversion, or apprehension, to an overt panic reaction in which the infant appears terrified, screams aloud, and turns away from the stranger, burying his head in his mother's breast. This "reaction to strangers," "eight-month anxiety," or "stranger anxiety" was found to have tremendous variations in timing, quantity, and quality by Margaret S. Mahler and her collaborators (1975) and this was even observed in the classic film on stranger anxiety by Spitz and Wolf.

A second reaction is well-known to psychoanalysts as *separation anxiety*. This is revealed when mother absents herself from the child's perceptual field. These two phenomena were originally considered by Freud and R.A. Spitz to be based on one "dynamic," that is, the infant's fear of loss or abandonment by mother. Subsequent research has introduced further refinements which need not be gone into in this book, and which Schecter mentions as well as Mahler (1975).

During the second year, there are behavioral developments which indicate that the child not only can discriminate and selectively value his mother, but that he has begun to represent her mentally, according to Schecter, with qualities of increasing *permanence* and objectivity.

> The evidence for the achievement of "object constancy" in this psychoanalytic sense—in contrast to the purely cognitive "object permanence" of *Piaget*—is rather fluid and reversible achievement and there are behaviors that would indicate that mother is represented mentally and invested with intense affect (Schecter, 1968).

Schecter states that in the third to the fifth years of life, the child begins to abstract and generalize the up-to-now largely concrete family members, roles, and situations. From the egocentric assumption of the one-to-one "me-you" situations, there is said to emerge a growing and momentous awareness that there are mommies, daddies, and children amongst whom the particular child is only one. Schecter continues to suggest that the child can now conceive a higher level interpersonal world, that is the triangular "I, you, and the others." The developing child grasps the fact that in the new cognitive-affective scheme of things, it becomes more and more evident, often too painfully, that mommy is no longer "all mine." The achievement of the triangular interpersonal world constitutes a new potential shattering of a developing self-identity. As

Schecter formulates this, the juvenile now knows: "I am no longer the exclusively loved and admired one to mother (or to father); brothers, sisters, father can have her too." But, this development is said to constitute the ground for moving into a social group and eventually valuing one's peers as one had previously valued one's parents. One can conceive of the development of the child's growing cognitive-affective capacity to conceive truly and experience the triangular interpersonal world as a crucial step in the master of social reality.

THE LEARNING OF CULTURAL PRESCRIPTIONS FOR OVERT BEHAVIOR

Sullivan claimed that the widespread practice of *telling* or reading *stories* to the child was another strong influence in transmitting certain of society's cultural prescriptions to the child. There are in general two types. One type may designate socially approved moral tales which have become ingrained in the culture because they embody complex ethical ideals in a fashion that can be grasped by a child. During Sullivan's generation, Bible stories, for example, might be read to the child before he reached the traditional age for starting formal schooling, at least in more literate homes. If one happens to grow in a cultural milieu where storytelling is a frequent form of entertainment, then the parent may tell such stories.

Sullivan is not entirely clear about the second type of storytelling or reading. He says they are inventions of the authority figure which may actually be pretty far from the socially approved moral stories and be a very special function of the parent personality. Thus, the child is said to be apt to be particularly impressed by long continued stories in which a parent takes the trouble to carry the imaginary protagonists night after night through new adventures. But, Sullivan does not specify any such stories. Since Sullivan grew in a culture where storytelling was then a frequent form of entertainment, as well as singing and dancing, we venture to suggest a few possible illustrations. They might be "ghost stories," some of which, as we now know, had an almost uncanny resemblance to some of C.G. Jung's archetypes. Or, they might embody mythical pagan themes. Or still again, they might be celebrations of famous folk heroes of Northern Ireland before the British brought civilization to the barbarian Irish: the O'Neils, the O'Donnells, and a great many more chieftains enshrined in Irish school books. Such stories were often not in harmony with the morality and theology of the Irish church.

In this fashion, according to Sullivan, children got the impression that they should be governed by certain influences, called values or judgments, or the ethical worth of certain types of behavior. Doubtless, the student who has grown during the reign of television and comic books will consider the practices which Sullivan refers to as archaic.

What Sullivan was driving at is this: these values, which children acquire as previously described, are experienced in the parataxic mode, that is, roughly, they are are non-logical, non-factual and virtually incapable of analysis. Hence, they do not necessarily coincide with the parents' observed behavior. This sort of phenomenon is somewhat analogous to the behavior of a parent who repeatedly tells his offspring that it is morally wrong to lie (or steal, as the case may be) while day after day he lies while talking to a neighbor in the child's presence.

But, often these values persist in "noteable" magic detachment from the child's actual living experience. Sullivan asserts that these values are apt to be rich soil for the production of verbalisms and that these verbalisms, because they are *derived from moral stories* or the like, which are part of the cultural heritage, have an effect on impressing the other person which is quite magical. And, just as a child approaching the juvenile era may not question the observed discrepancy between what he is told he ought to do, or not to do, and the behavior of the authority figure, he learns to develop a very important discrimination between what can be expressed or demonstrated and that which cannot. The latter has to be relegated to covert processes in contrast to the overt. The discrepancy between what must be relegated to *covert processes* and what can be *overt* becomes very puzzling to the child. He has a natural need for information about all sorts of things, but in some mysterious fashion they are taboo. So, he resorts to asking ostensibly rational questions about various sorts of things such as, why the parents do this and that in the morning when, for example, he merely wants to know why "mother and father do not say a word to each other when they wake to begin the day." Summarily, he may resort to asking pointless questions, questions which *conceal* what he wants to know. And he may go on from there to asking repetitive, as well as pointless questions, an autistic combination of words which "refers" to what the child really wants to know. To the parents, he may seem to make a virtue of questioning for questioning's sake—which may in fact become a form of malicious mischief. And eventually, all of this may seem quite rational because the questioning has a patina of rational curiosity.

THE GROWING NECESSITY FOR DISTINGUISHING BETWEEN REALITY AND FANTASY

It is a well-known fact that children have a considerable need for parents' participation in *childhood play*, at least as an attentive audience, and if possible, as people who perform a role, unless there are siblings who serve this purpose. Unfortunately, a good many children, for one reason or another, do not have an audience. A child in this category is lonely, and loneliness can be a foreshadowing of the far greater loneliness which appears during pre-adolescence. Subsequently, the lonely child, according to Sullivan, has a very rich fantasy life. In other words, his mind creates imaginary personifications which will influence his behavior. It does not follow that the young child recognizes fantasy *per se*. He has learned a lot about the reality of a cup or spoon or his favorite toys.

It is important here to mention Piaget's famous studies of children's gradually developing powers to abstract and generalize. The child is well acquainted with the concrete objects of his daily existence. On the other hand, the creations of the child's mind may be just as real to him as a cup and spoon. Moreover, many things that are perfectly real to the child are very heavily invested with autistic, referential (thought) processes by the child. Hence, there is an indefinitely great area of life for the child where fantasy and reality are indistinguishable. Of course, the interests of adults have little or no significance to the child. Toys are said to be very useful to the very young child for the purpose of exercising newly matured abilities: "they do not have any of those relationships which cause us to carry collision damage on automobiles." The distinction between what anyone would agree was real and what is "unutterably the child's own" imaginary, fantastic possession is of no particular interest to the adults.

These ideas of Sullivan gain consensual validation by Mahler's observations on the individual Patterning of Rapproachment that the toddler achieves at the twenty-first month of development, the optimal distance from the mothering one by using several dynamisms.

1. The development of language in terms of naming objects and expressing desires with specific words.
2. The so called "internalization" process which could be inferred both from act of "identification" with this good-providing mother and father and from the internalization of rules and demands (beginnings of super ego).
3. Progress in the ability to express wishes and fantasies through symbolic play as well as the use of play for mastery (Schecter, 1968).

However, by the end of childhood, when the child has reached the age of approximately five years, the pressure toward socialization becomes very great; that is, in part, the carefully sorting out of that which is capable of being agreed to by the authority figure. This carefully sorting out is the first "very vivid" manifestation in life of the role of consensual validation. In its simplest meaning, *consensual validation* is merely a consensus between two people that can be reached, as to what something is, or what it means, or whether it is true. In its most sophisticated forms, it applies to mathematics and natural science.

Sullivan stated that consensually validated symbols underlie almost all operations in the syntaxic mode. In early infancy, all of the baby's experiences are "global," apparently possessing no clear-cut distinctions regarding such things as time and space, I and Thou, etc. In mid or late infancy, he starts to make elementary discriminations in his experiences. But, they are not logically or factually connected; there is no movement of one idea to its logical successor. Experiences are associated in patterns.

The symbols which refer to parataxic experience are very poor instruments for understanding the world, even though most adults probably employ them more than they know when they engage in abstract thought. For example, at the present time, as one listens to people comment on political and economic problems, one is startled at the lack of clear logical thinking, or respect for facts. Given Sullivan's preoccupation with interpersonal relations, he emphasized that what distinguishes syntaxic operations from everything else that goes on in the mind is that they can, under appropriate circumstances, work quite precisely with other people.

> And the only reason that they come to work quite precisely with other people is that in actual contact with other people there has been some degree of exploration, analysis and the obtaining of information (Sullivan, 1953).

In *Personal Psychopathology*, Sullivan (1953) stated that consensually valid information is the result of a *conscious* education of relations discriminated on multiple bases of experience with other people and things. This is a way of saying that logical, rational thinking is a social, cooperative enterprise.

Failures at Socialization

The business of socializing the child so that what the parents call purely imaginary events are not actually true or have not actually happened is said to be so important that it is enforced by the end of childhood on practically everyone. Sullivan asserted that the lonelier the child has been, the more striking may be his need of continuous recall and foresight in order to distinguish and "fix" in his mind the distinctions conventionally regarded as having happened (whether five seconds ago, a year ago, or a millenium) and what was part of fantasy processes. In the next era, the juvenile may make "shocking" mistakes and get himself laughed at by his more erudite classmates or playmates, or punished for his reporting what adults call lively fantasy as real. The threat of such a fate can in itself be very disconcerting to a lonely child who has a bent toward *social isolation*. This is one of many more or less circular processes that are poignantly familiar to clinicians. The *lonely child* already has had to develop a rich fantasy life in lieu of an audience and participation by the authority figures. As a result, even if he possesses outstanding intellectual capacity, he is likely to be relatively slow and wooden when he needs to make a very rapid discrimination between what is his private fantasy and what may be consensually validated. This lack, in turn, enhances the vulnerability of the lonely child, once he enters the juvenile era, to ridicule, punishment, and whatever other devices some juveniles may create in order to increase their amusement at the victim's expense. Not surprisingly, such experiences tend to give the helpless juvenile a feeling of risk in life. A partial arrest of development occurs because the lonely youngster may withdraw as best he can from intercourse with his peers and therefore fails to learn or to learn adequately certain "dynamisms" that are normally acquired during the juvenile era. Of course, if he is not utterly crushed, he may become a whiz in mathematics, provided he has the necessary intellectual capacity. In such a case, he may, if he is very gifted, eventually become a professor of math. On the other hand, if he is of ordinary intelligence, he may fail to learn either scholastic, social or occupational skills. It may happen (it has happened) when the school authorities once release him from what is to him a particular form of hell, he secures a job as a messenger boy, for example, and when he grows a few years older, a job as a service elevator operator which, if he is fortunate, he keeps for the rest of his life. Depending largely on the parental background, he may be forever isolated sexually from men or women.

THE JUVENILE ERA

In Sullivanian psychology, the various eras are not biologically or socially fixed. However, no one doubts that in a given society there is a progression from infancy to what is conventionally defined as maturity. In *Personal Psychopathology* (1953) Sullivan wrote:

> The clearness with which these stages of personality growth may be distinguished diminishes as we proceed from the intra-uterine condition onward. For obvious reasons, individuals in each succeeding stage show more or less striking differentiation because of dissimilar experience, and each individual becomes progressively more individuated. For this reason the application of any schematization of individuals in the juvenile era (and preadolescence) and thereafter, is (or are) anything but all-encompassing—which is perhaps not too bad, after all.

The maturation of the need for peers "ushers in" the juvenile era, which in the United States is roughly synonymous with the beginning of formal schooling. It happens that much of childhood life is egocentric. In the well-to-do classes, especially, children are not infrequently put in an educative situation before they have passed through this phase of their development. One can frequently observe egocentric speech. Sullivan asserted that by late childhood children's speech has become a great field for play and a very considerable aid in one's fantasy life, so that in a nursery school they can apparently talk a blue streak to one another, but the talk is not truly "interactional" or transactional.

As childhood progresses, a time is said to be reached when there is a very rapid acceleration of change in the character of fantasy. This change is directed toward "burying, losing interest in, forgetting, or modifying what may in very early childhood have been truly incredibly fantastic imaginary playmates," toward an attempt to personify playmates like oneself. Now the child starts to have rather realistic imaginary playmates. "Now they begin to be as like him as can be..." (Sullivan, 1953). Within very real limits, this is reminiscent of Freud's ideas on childhood amnesia, except for the latter, forgetting is particularly a repression of sexual fantasies. Ernest Schachtel (1959) has provided a very provocative formulation of childhood amnesia, although it has not received wide acceptance and will bear careful study. School introduces one to the great world outside the home, with all its virtues and shortcomings. Hence, it is the time for becoming social—which will be presently spelled out. But, it is a very crucial phase of development, if any one era can be thus meaningfully characterized. People who "bog down" in the juvenile era, owing to previous unfortunate experience, have a very conspicuous disqualification for a comfortable way of life.

Sullivan claimed that the *juvenile era* is the first developmental stage in which the limitations and peculiarities of the home as a socializing influence begin to be open to remedy unless it is underminded by forces mentioned below. Sullivan wrote:

> In this culture, where education is compulsory, it is the school society that rectifies or modifies in the juvenile era a great deal of the unfortunate direction of personality evolution conferred upon the young by their parents and others constituting the family group (Sullivan, 1953).

One wishes that he had also dwelt on the limitations and peculiarities of the school. Even if teachers were paragons—and Sullivan had no illusions about that—they are often hemmed in by parents, school administrators, and perhaps above all by the formidable school board, often comprised of people who are in no way qualified to evaluate school programs and procedures and its frequently ambitious superintendent of schools. There are variations in the school set-up which cannot adequately be discussed in this book.

In the cities of the East and West coasts of the United States, racial conflict has frequently been an enormously disruptive force, which is more or less glossed over by the media. Unhappily, every so often, some outrageous deed takes place and it cannot always be ignored by the media. Some older boy will decide to enhance his education by raping the young female teacher in one of the school corridors. Or, he may vent his spleen on some male teacher who has reprimanded him for misbehavior by plunging a switchblade knife into him. But, there are other more subtle influences that often tend to limit *formal schooling*. In working class and lower middle class neighborhoods, the teacher, almost of necessity, given a class of more than 30 pupils, has to go through a set routine day after day. In this set-up, the teacher will depart from conventional values at his/her peril. Furthermore, in these schools education tends to be narrowly practical. Many working class and lower middle class students are not likely to aim at a college or university education, even if it is available. After all, in New York City, for example, garbage collectors, when one takes into consideration the "fringe benefits," pensions, as well as salaries which they receive, are probably better paid than most university professors or junior business executives. It seems to be chiefly in the Upper Middle and Upper Classes that first class schools are found.

Therefore, one has to exercise some discrimination when one writes about schools. They vary enormously in the United States and throughout the world. And the social life of the pupils of the various classes mentioned in a brief and loose fashion also varies enormously. "Social accommodation" among juveniles who live in one neighborhood varies significantly from that of juveniles from another.

Possible Changes in the Self-System

In *Conceptions of Modern Psychiatry*, Sullivan (1953) wrote that the peculiarity of the *self-system* is that as it grows it functions, in accordance with its state of development, right from the start. This implies that the *self dynamism* or *self-system* once it takes on a particular organization retains it fairly rigidly throughout life. But in subsequent years Sullivan (1953) apparently tried to modify this idea. In *The Interpersonal Theory of Psychiatry*, he wrote:

> It is in general true that, as one passes over one of these more-or-less determinable thresholds of a developmental era, everything that has gone before becomes reasonably open to influence; this is true even in the organization of the self-system, which as I suppose I cannot stress too much, is remarkably inclined to maintain its direction. The changes which take place at the thresholds of the developmental eras, as outlined here,

may be far-reaching; they touch upon much of what has already been acquired as personality, often making it somewhat acutely inadequate, or at any rate not fully relevant for the sudden new expanding of the personal horizon. Thus the beginning phase of a developmental era may considerably affect those inappropriate aspects of personality which emerge from what the person has undergone up to then.

Essentially Sullivan leaves plenty of room for personality growth, for change and — of necessity — for retrogression. One of the most important variables pertaining to limitations of self-development is *social*. In *Personal Psychopathology*, Sullivan (1953) was bitterly critical of American society. The book was written at the beginning of the Great Depression when great masses (millions) of the American people suffered incredible social and personal hardship. However, Sullivan lectured with an eye toward mental disorders or "difficulties in living." Knowing that his death was not very far off, he strove to improve what he regarded as the sad state of American psychiatry within an inevitably brief time span.

Stratification and Social Accommodation

The following quotation from Arthur M. Schlesinger, Jr., the noted historian, throws considerable light on modern Western man's personal insecurity.

> Our modern industrial economy, based on impersonality, interchangeability and speed, has worn away the old protective securities without creating new ones. It has failed to develop an organizational framework of its own within which self-realization on a large scale is possible. Freedom in industrial society, as a result, has a negative rather than a positive connotation. It means a release from external restraints rather than a deep and abiding sense of self-control and purpose (Green, 1952).

The division of labor has an important bearing on the self in modern society. The sociologist Arnold W. Green has pointed out that the division of labor is an arrangement found in all societies whereby people perform different tasks at the same time, and exchange their economic surpluses in a formal or informal way. The division of labor is said to be not only universal but is also the common basis for stratification, by which people are ranked in higher and lower positions. Green calls attention to the fact that in all societies some people obey, while others are obeyed. There are those who defer while others are deferred to.

It is the fact that during the *juvenile era* young people are directly introduced to some of the hard necessities of *social stratification* which we wish to stress. But, it should be mentioned, that even before they enter school, children often observe how their parents rank on the block in which they live because the parents betray it in the way they talk, with whom they talk, how they defer to some and condescend toward others.

Children may notice whether they live in a house of their own or in a tenement. The location of the block itself is also significant. As we know, children listen to their parents talk. They notice that some people are mentioned with respect, others casually, and still others with indifference if not contempt. Even in the Medical establishment Foreign Medical Graduates (FMG's) are ranked according to their countries of origin.

According to Green (1952), *"stratification"*

> is universal because it is necessary. All group activity must be organized, which means that authority to direct this or that operation must be either assumed or delegated. Society, and the groups which make up society, reward those with the responsibility of directing others, and of supervising an operation through to its completion, with authority, respect, fame and/or wealth. Those who do not direct others but merely work at some routine task are rewarded when they do their job better than others with whom they cooperate and compete — with at least appreciation, and in most cases with money or some other material reward.

However, Green points out, that it is the division of labor in modern industrial society that must be elaborately stratified. He reinforces this observation by calling attention to the fact that the assembly line and the corporate organization which controls it require thousands of men to perform different specialties in order to produce and distribute a single pair of shoes. A line of command is necessary to ensure that the workers perform their individual tasks in a vast integrated operation that the majority cannot even visualize. "Although current political ideology denies this, the fact remains that modern industrial society creates a greater *range* of social inequality than the world has ever known" (Green, 1952).

Has it ever occurred to the reader to wonder why children are required to attend school? Those of us who like children have observed them with a touch of sadness. The normal child's delight in play seems endless, his energy boundless, his trust in his small world often abundant. Are they required by the state to attend school in order to learn and appreciate the best that man has thought and said and done? The causes of compulsory school attendance are complex. Sullivan, despite his extraordinary understanding of people, clung to the Liberal tradition which holds that only through formal education can one develop his capacities, intellectual, moral and so forth.

One reason that children are required to attend school is that they must learn various skills if they are to survive in modern industrial society. There is no question about that. The fact that, owing to complex historical events, droves of youngsters wander the streets of the city lacking in any useful skill or perhaps a desire even to learn is not a happy turn of affairs for the United States. They are a danger to themselves and to society. But, the reason for compulsory school attendance (which is not quite so compulsory as it was in the days when a delinquent student feared the Truant Officer) that concerns us more directly is that in school the pupil begins to learn *social accommodation*. Sullivan (1953) is very clear about that. He said:

> In almost all cases, however, the more emphatically effective contribution of the juvenile era is that of *social accommodation* —that is, a simply astounding broadening of the grasp of how many slight differences in living there are; how many of these differences seem to be all right, even if pretty new; and how many of them don't seem to be right, but nonetheless how unwise one is to attempt to correct them.

The school years are said to be a time when a degree of crudeness in interpersonal relations, very rarely paralleled in later years, is the rule. Nevertheless, Sullivan immediately adds that the opportunity which is laid before the young juvenile for catching on to how other people are looked upon by authority figures and by each other is an exceedingly important part of the educative process. Thus, the amount of education, in the broad sense, that comes from the juvenile era is "immensely important." As the juvenile's life progresses he can see what other juveniles are doing—either what they are

> getting away with, or being reproved for—and can notice differences between people which he had never conceived of, because previously he had had nothing whatever on which to base an idea of something different from his own experience (Sullivan, 1953).

Social Subordination

There is a great change in the type of authority, and in the kind of authority in the juvenile era. According to Sullivan, by requiring formal education, the social order provides a succession of new authority figures "who are often fortunate in their impersonality." Be that as it may, he fails to stress the fact that formal education provides a discipline which will make it possible for millions of people to fit into a modern impersonal economy, whether it be capitalistic, socialistic, or whatever. In any case, Sullivan asserts that in his relations with his teacher and other authority figures "such as the assistant principal" (the principal may be such a lofty figure that he is ordinarily beyond the reach of the juvenile), the juvenile is expected to do things on demand. Compliance, non-compliance, or rebellion will earn rewards or punishments. One might add that the authority figures generally act within socially defined rules and limits. This is a matter which has broad implications that go far beyond the scope of this book.

ACCOMMODATION AND COMPETITION

In the *Conceptions of Modern Psychiatry*, Sullivan (1953) wrote that the child proceeds into the juvenile era by virtue of a new tendency toward cooperation, to doing things in *accommodation* to the personality of others. Green defines cooperation as the continuous and common endeavor of two or more persons to perform a task or to reach a goal that is commonly cherished. Whether the goal, psychologically speaking, need always be commonly cherished is debatable. It usually is, but it need not be. According to Green (1952), in any concrete situation, competition and cooperations are, in varying proportions, always included. He distinguishes *primary cooperation* from *secondary cooperation*. Primary cooperation entails a virtual fusion of the individual in the group. The group is said to contain all or nearly all of each individual's life. "There is an interlocking identification of individual, group and task performed." Cooperation is so highly prized that means and goals become one. The Israeli Kibbutz is an illuminating example of this fusion. There is a certain resemblance between Green's notion of primary cooperation and Erich Fromm's notion of "primary ties" in *Escape From Freedom*. But there are also vital differences. The primary ties (where the person experiences himself only as a member of a clan or tribe — not as an individual) which bind a primitive group or a present day preliterate group are characteristic of man's upward rise toward individuation "in the historical process" which Fromm interprets according to Marx, who was indebted to Hegel. For Green, Marx's and Fromm's metaphysical interpretation of an historical process is sheer speculation which will not stand up under close logical analysis. Green's illustration is illuminating. Thus, he writes, that an example of primary cooperation is the daily routine of life in a monastery. Only a dogmatist would assert that the traditional routine of life in a Cistercian monastery is primitive, historically, sociologically, or whatever. Whether there is much primary cooperation left in Western society is another question. In recent years, various student groups, and young non-student people have attempted to experiment with communities governed by primary cooperation. Unlike the Israeli Kibbutz, they have all failed after a brief period. The contemporary world leaves little room for the dedication, simplicity, self-discipline and unworldliness of primary cooperation.

As for *secondary cooperation*, we are all directly or indirectly familiar with it. It is part of the life of a factory, an automobile plant, or the beehive network of offices in a modern corporation. It transcends the capitalist economy in any highly industrialized society. Hence, modern economic "progress" is always bought at a price, and a person who harbors utopian fantasies of some future society in which its members will abandon greed, love one another, develop various potentialities for which the market has no value, and joyfully cooperate for the common good might re-examine the realities of social life. Green has stated some of the characteristics of secondary cooperation. Whether others before him or after him have not said the same is of no importance for the purposes of this book.

> Secondary cooperation is highly formalized and specialized, and each individual devotes only part of his life to the group which is held together with it. Cooperation is not itself a value; attitudes are more likely to be individualistic and calculating. Most members of the group feel some loyalty toward the group, but the welfare of the group is not their first consideration....Each performs his task, and thus helps the others to perform their tasks, so that he can *separately* enjoy the fruits of his cooperation (Green, 1952).

It is in and out of the classroom, in the school yard, or the athletic field that the juvenile is educated ("socialized") in such a fashion that in days to come he will be able to become a self-supporting member of his society, and add his share or play the necessary roles for its maintenance. It is a tribute to Sullivan's ability that, although he had no great intellectual penetration of socio-economic processes, he intuitively grasped the psychological dynamisms which "mold" the youngster for a status and role in adult society. However, there is a significant shift in emphasis regarding cooperation from *Conceptions of Modern Psychiatry* to *The Interpersonal Theory of Psychiatry* where it is clarified at some length.

Competition

In numerous lectures, especially in the series *Conceptions of Modern Psychiatry* (1953), Sullivan, who usually delivered his "talks" to a psychiatric audience, took competition, cooperation, and compromise for granted, which one can observe as typical of children in the early school years, outstanding developments of the juvenile era. Yet, he believed that one does not really know something unless one can state its meaning clearly to another. Although he had a profound and very refined interest in the fine arts, Sullivan seemed to think that aesthetic ideas were incapable of formulation, particularly in words. At the time of his death, he was attempting to develop his ideas in a more systematic fashion. Because of a gravely impaired heart, he knew his life span would be relatively short. (Probably for that reason, his lectures are urgent, frequently incomplete, and sometimes contain ideas that are obscure.) Yet, in the United States, he seems to have been by far the most influential American psychiatrist. And his influence is growing, despite the obscurities, which apparently have not amounted to much in the face of his achievements. Parenthetically there are not a few obscurities in the writings of Freud, but a number of psychiatrists we have read during the past generation, after genuflecting before them, pass on to more workable conceptions — Freudian or otherwise. Thanks to the rapid growth of psychology and psychiatry during the past 20 years, a psychoanalyst may now diverge from the master without an introductory homage.

In discussing the characteristics of the various eras, we are discussing ongoing, developing processes, not finished results at least until one has reached maturity. Unfortunately, for causes which we hope to make clear, both idiosyncratic and interpersonal or social factors sometimes intervene and destroy some cherished hope, or some rapidly growing ability, until, as Sullivan might say, the individual becomes an inferior caricature of what he might have been. Some social convention may be so inert and blind that it crushes many a promising career or some rare and precious talent.

Again, because we know no better reliable authority to fill in some minor gaps that Sullivan left behind him, we will quote Green's (1952) definition of competition. "In competition, two or more parties strive for the same goal which none is prepared or expected to share with the others." It differs from conflict, in that it stops short of coercion. Of course, Sullivan is concerned with personal competition, not with business or political competition. According to the latter, the juvenile society itself encourages competitive efforts of all kinds. Sullivan believed that such competition is "natural" but, in a society where, within limits, the economy is governed by competition, the authority figures encourage competition. And this is outstandingly true of the United States and Western society in general. Interestingly, the communist countries have introduced their own brands of competition, which, according to reports, can be pretty fierce — despite their official ideologies. Individually (and socially), competition may become destructive. Sullivan (1953) has stated this clearly.

> In what I call chronically juvenile people one sees a competitive way of life in which nearly everything that has real importance is part of a process of getting ahead of the other fellow. And if there is also a malevolent transformation of personality, getting the other fellow down becomes the outstanding pattern in the integration of interpersonal relations.

Sullivan thought that American society (and unfortunately this is true of contemporary American society) was prevailingly juvenile. However, one must note that no society can exist without a minimum of cooperation and compromise.

Compromise

Although Sullivan pointed out that *compromise*, like competition, is invariably enforced by the juvenile society itself or the juvenile authorities and is a very necessary addition to one's equipment for living with one's fellows, he does not stress it in his theoretical formulations. But, he did not neglect it in his clinical lectures. To compromise, he used to say, is to give up part of what one wants in order to obtain the rest. Obviously, compromise entails a nice equation, and unless governed by two or more persons, mutual respect and consideration can easily shift in the direction of submission or domination. It is a mark of profound insecurity to be willing to yield almost everything, as it is equally so if one is always trying to yield nothing. Whether there are matters on which one should never compromise is a nice philosophical question that must be passed over.

CONTROL OF FOCAL AWARENESS

Sullivan claimed that the juvenile era is the time when the world begins to be really complicated by the presence of other people. Thus far in life the child's world is directly complicated by his transection of only one or two institutions: the school and perhaps the religious institution. Sullivan followed the psychoanalytic tradition of ignoring (when he was not attacking) the importance of the Church, whether for good or ill. In view of the fact that in the Western tradition, religion has been the source of morality, this omission is serious. Sullivanian psychology is essentially social psychology and, therefore, the omission cannot be explained away. If there is not commonly held and commonly shared *morality*, no common or shared possession of *shoulds* and *should not's*, what is to hold society together? And since doctrinal religion seems to be rapidly declining, what will the source of a shared morality be?

Leaving aside the profoundly important question of compromise we take up the topic of the control of focal awareness. The "full educational effort" of the school is said to be addressed to the extinction of the autistic from the expressed thought and other behavior of the juvenile. Sullivan held that this learning of successful ways of expression and successful types of performance covers so much ground and receives so much encouragement from all sorts of educative influences, ranging from anxiety to carefully awarded prestige with one's fellows, that by the end of the eighth grade, if not earlier, a person of normal endowment has given up a great many of the ideas and operations, which, in childhood, and in the home, were all right. The effect of this learning is so powerful that whatever is not perfectly appropriate or easily modified to meet the criteria of the school, becomes virtually erased from consciousness. While the American school is assuredly not dominated by a rigid ideology as is the case in communist Russia, it is geared toward the creation of a good citizen who can take his place, whatever it may turn out to be, in a modern industrial society. How well and intelligently it accomplishes this task is another question.

It is the increasing power of the self-system which has been "shaped" with the help of language to *control focal awareness*, that makes possible the abandoning of the ideas and operations of childhood. Let the reader imagine any one of numerous occasions when he temporarily relinquished this control and allowed his thoughts and fantasies to float more or less freely. Then perhaps he will have a better understanding of the ability of the self from which the juvenile era onward increasingly controls the things we attend to. Chiefly owing to their immaturity, many juveniles can be cruel. But their cruelty is quite crude and superficial in comparison with the cruelty of adults who, because of their knowledge and skill in interpersonal relations, can inflict "psychic" wounds on the other with finesse and a knowledge of the other person's vulnerable traits. We would like to point out vis-à-vis the therapist the danger of cruel manipulation of patients that may occur in therapy. In any case, the direct, crude, and critical reactions of his peers to the autistic language behavior or unconventional actions of some hapless juvenile not yet weaned from the life of childhood can alert him to the demands of his altered situation and compel him to adopt the required speech and behavior patterns. Moreover, the speech, behavior patterns and demands of the teachers and administrators, are "relatively formulable and predictable." Thus, they tend to introduce an element of order and objectivity in the juvenile's experience which may have been previously rather tenuous.

Sullivan (1953) claimed,

> In other words, the juvenile has extraordinary opportunity to learn a great deal about security operations, to learn ways of being free from anxiety, in terms of comparatively understandable sanctions and their violations. . . And insofar as the sanctions and the operations which will avoid anxiety make sense, can be consensually validated, the self-system effectively controls focal awareness so that what does not make sense tends to get no particular attention.

Anxiety serves as an effective instrumentality of the self to "shepherd" effective manifestations of consciousness to occur more or less in the syntaxic mode — "the mode of experience which offers some possibility of predicting the novel, and some possibility of real interpersonal communication."

Control of focal awareness implies that one attends, or can attend, to things going on in one's mind or in the world that do matter. But many people—perhaps everyone to some degree—misuse selective inattention so that one ignores things that do matter. And one ignores things that do matter in interpersonal relations—and often with regard to very abstract but important matters—because they make one feel uncomfortable or anxious. Sometimes they make one fearful as well.

SUBLIMATION

In various contexts, we have referred to *sublimation* or what Sullivan called the sublimatory reformulation of patterns of behavior and covert processes (attitudes, motives, emotions, thoughts, etc.) He claimed that the educative process which is tributary to success in living is very largely a manifestation of sublimation, not of rational analysis and valid formulation. This kind of educative process, in contrast to the learning of mathematics, covers "a very great deal of one's education for living." When sublimation works, it works beautifully but it must not be "overloaded." Thus, a patient who is a gifted painter discovered that whenever he is engaged in intense sexual relations he can not paint and vice versa. To what degree one can sublimate sexual drives, hateful tendencies, competitive drives, perhaps even love, which the contemporary world does not seem to foster, will probably vary from individual to individual and his particular life circumstances. But any intense, energy laden drive has indefinitely specifiable limits, beyond which a sublimatory reformulation breaks down.

Insofar as sublimation is not overloaded, Sullivan (1953) taught, it

> gives one great surety in what one is doing; and one's certainty is not even disturbed by the fact that somebody else may reason better to a different end. Thus, when a juvenile acquires a pattern of relating himself to someone else which works and is approved, he simply *knows* that what he is doing is right. And this certainty comes about because there is, in the juvenile era, an increasing power of the self-system to control the contents of awareness, and because the acquisition of the pattern is itself unwitting. Since there is no particular reason for anyone to try to bring into the juvenile's awareness how he arrived at these reformulations of behavior, most of us come into adult life with a great many firmly entrenched ways of dealing with our fellow man which we cannot explain adequately. . . People are not even particularly vulnerable to inquiry in this area, because, by the time anybody is apt to be investigating it, they have a whole variety of devices for heading off awkwardness.

SUPERVISORY PATTERNS OF THE SELF

An almost inevitable outcome of the most fortunate kind of juvenile experience is said to be the appearance of *supervisory patterns* of the self. In certain instances, they are virtually sub-personifications ("subpersonalities"), or imaginary people who are always with us. During the juvenile era, these supervisory patterns are born and develop. With some refinements they persist—and may grow for many years, sometimes with considerable requirements. The one most familiar to the reader is probably what Freud called the Super-Ego. In the traditional home, one is taught that certain things are morally right and others are morally wrong. Such teachings, in the past, have been part of religion. If one attends a parochial school, such teachings will be elaborated and refined. In the opinion of many, the Bible is still considered the greatest source of moral enlightenment. However, in much contemporary literature both popular and otherwise, the notion of morality is radically watered down so that the criteria of what sometimes passes for morality are either obscure or specious, as is the case with hedonism. Hedonism does not make good sense regardless of one's liking for cherries and cherry blossoms in the spring.

But there are several less famous supervisory patterns. It is not *comme il faut* to scratch oneself in public. Sometimes a person will absentmindedly start to scratch some part of his body and then an internal process intervenes to remind him, as it were, that he is being observed by others. And so he may try to cover up his "mistake" by pretending he is trying to brush the dust off his coat or pants. The supervisory pattern which intervened is call the *Spectator*. The spectator is an unobstructive but very observant fellow who diligently observes what one "shows" to and does with others. In these days when so many people seem eager to show everything, it is not easy to provide illustrations. Traditionally, one would be careful to walk in a dignified manner, neither slouching nor walking as if one were flat-footed. There was a time—though it may seem like ancient history—when girls did not "show" their slip or any other undergarment. An "accident" which revealed some part of a dainty undergarment could be very embarrassing. These illustrations are somewhat superficial, but they indicate the reason for an appropriate Spectator to keep one on the *qui vivre*. Moreover, what one may "show" as a member of a lower social class may differ from what is permissible among the upper classes.

A writer of any integrity always has a supervisory pattern called *The Reader*, who, so to speak, looks over one's shoulder when one writes—unless one becomes very weary and intellectually sluggish. The reader observes such things as style, lucidity of presentation, appropriateness of grammar, etc. Sullivan's reader became so "paranoid" that he was virtually unable to write during the latter part of his career.

If one lectures in public, one has a supervisory pattern called the *Hearer*. He is "strikingly competent" in judging the relevancy of what one is talking about. He observes the clarity of what one is saying.

Similarly, one's grammar is scrutinized. Perhaps he pays careful attention to how well one "projects" one's lecture.

In general, these supervisory patterns can be rigorous or "permissive." At present, American society seems to drift toward loose standards in almost every area of life, not least of which is television.

THE LEARNING OF DISPARAGEMENT

In many of his lectures Sullivan talked about a behavior pattern which seems to be widespread throughout the United States, namely, the technique of *disparaging*, belittling others in a wholesale fashion in order to reduce the stature of others. This behavior pattern, he claimed, is based on the principle that if one feels only as high as a molehill there shall be no mountains around one.

Due to morbidity of parental security operations, the juvenile may be taught to disparage others. For example, the parental morbid security operations may occur because one or both parents feel threatened by the revealing nature of juvenile communication and consequently disparage teachers and others with whom they feel compared. When the juvenile learns the "disparaging business," it generalizes. One must remember that almost every day and every night the juvenile is subjected to the parental morbidity. One can hardly imagine a more self-destructive tendency. Since one learns to be human, or fully human, from learning numerous attributes or traits and behavior patterns of others, if one is surrounded by animals or sub-human monsters, how can one learn to be a person endowed with the worth and dignity of a human being? Unwittingly, the juvenile gradually becomes entrapped in a principle of living that may be formulated as "I am the best of swine." And thus, the disparagement business strikes at the roots of that which is essentially human, namely, the utterly vital and essential role of interpersonal relations. Parents who are so morbid that they undermine all human decency pass on to their offspring attitudes which, barring great good fortune in subsequent eras of personality development, guarantee that their children will be psychologically crippled.

Sullivan, of course, knew that, in general, morbid interpersonal relations are expressions or manifestations of "morbidities" in "the culture." A generation after Sullivan lived and lectured, there have developed deep lying social morbidities which even he, far sighted in so many ways, could scarcely imagined. In what great American city did the reader recently take a long leisurely stroll on some lovely summer night?

THE CONCEPTION OF ORIENTATION IN LIVING

Various writers have employed the notion of a "well-integrated personality" to characterize a healthy mature human being who can "adjust" to the circumstances of his milieu intelligently and with a reasonable measure of satisfaction with life. However, this entire notion is somewhat vague. Sullivan's *conception of orientation in living* is quite clear though it does not seem to have been much appreciated. In order to appreciate its usefulness, the reader can always ask himself, how well do I fulfill these criteria? It reads as follows:

> One is oriented in living to the extent to which one has formulated, or can easily be led to formulate (or has insight into), data of the following types: the integrating tendencies (needs) which customarily characterize one's interpersonal relations; the circumstances appropriate to their satisfaction and relatively anxiety-free discharge; and the more or less remote goals for the approximation of which one will forego intercurrent opportunities for the satisfaction of the enhancement of one's prestige (Sullivan, 1953).

Of course, normally one's orientation in living becomes progressively broadened in subsequent eras. Sullivan claimed that to the extent that the juvenile knows, or could be easily be led to know, what needs motivate his relations with others, and under what circumstances these needs are appropriate and relatively apt to be fulfilled without damage to his self-respect, to this extent he has gotten a great deal "out of his first plunge into socialization." He will not sacrifice his integrity or his values for the sake of transient opportunities for having pleasure or "fun" or whatever. He has what in years gone by would be called "character." This development assumes the juvenile has had fortunate opportunity, such as a home where the parents are affectionate and reasonably wise in the ways of child rearing. He will have been sufficiently fortunate in his interpersonal relations to successfully negotiate the first three eras of development. But a great deal remains to be accomplished if he is going to be one of the lucky ones who arrive at maturity without serious problems.

REFERENCES

Ellenberger, H.F. *The Discovery of the Unconscious.* Basic Books, New York, 1970.

Erikson, E.H. *Childhood and Society.* W.W. Norton, New York, 1950.

Freud, S. *An Outline of Psychoanalysis.* W.W. Norton, New York, 1949.

Green, A.W. *Sociology.* McGraw-Hill, New York, 1952.

Lincourt, J.M., Olczak, P.V., Pierce, C.S., and Sullivan, H.S. on the human self. *Psychiat.* 1974; 1: 37:78–87.

Mahler, M.S. *The Psychological Birth of the Human Infant.* Basic Books, New York, 1975.

Mullahy, P. *Psychoanalysis and Interpersonal Psychiatry: The Contributions of Harry Stack Sullivan*. Science House, New York, 1970.

Schachtel, E.G. *Metamorphosis*. Basic Books, New York, 1959.

Schecter, D.E. The oedipus complex: Considerations of ego development and parental interaction. *Contemp. Psychoanal.* 1968; 4:111.

Stern, D. *The First Relationship*. Harvard Univ. Press, New York, 1975.

Sullivan, H.S. *Conceptions of Modern Psychiatry*. W.W. Norton, New York, 1953.

Sullivan, H.S. *The Interpersonal Theory of Psychiatry*. W.W. Norton, New York, 1953.

Sullivan, H.S. *Personal Psychopathology*. W.W. Norton, New York, 1972.

5

Preadolescence to Maturity

The juvenile era is "marked" by a need for peers, for playmates rather like oneself. *Preadolescence* is ushered in around the age of eight and one-half or nine and one-half by the appearance of a new type of interest in a *particular* person of the same sex who becomes a close friend or "chum." It seems very simple — simple to understand as a conception marking a given era of development and simple to achieve as a pattern of interpersonal relations. In the former case, the reader can easily grasp the distinction. As for the pattern of interpersonal relations the word *chum* signifies, it has often been ignored by psychologists and psychiatrists known to us. Of course, clever writers can still earn a fortune by writing popular books on love — or better still, love and sex. In past years, when Mullahy lectured on Sullivanian psychiatry to undergraduates, he discovered that they (especially females) confused preadolescent and adolescent *intimacy* with *romantic love*.

Hoping to clarify this confusion, we pointed out that in the words of John Dewey romantic love is as modern as big battleships. Love is not blind, but romantic "love" often is, and therein lies the problem. Sullivan (1953) states explicitly that in the type of preadolescent interpersonal relationships he had in mind, the chums are of the same sex, where "the other fellow takes on a perfectly novel relationship with the person concerned: he becomes of practically equal importance in all fields of value." This is a definition of intimacy, though it needs to be elaborated. However, apart from the intrinsic joy which this kind of intimacy brings about, it has to be regarded as a prelude to intimacy in heterosexual relationships among reasonably mature adults. *Preadolescent* chumship has no essential connection with sexuality, although, according to Sullivan, some members of preadolescent gangs may engage in sexual experimentation on the threshold of adolescence.

A large number of human societies have now been studied sufficiently to provide world-wide information on preadolescent sexual behavior at this particular developmental era. In a cross cultural study of sexual behavior of different societies in 1951, Clellan S. Ford and Frank A. Beach reported data that lends Sullivan's ideas consensual validation.

In order to clarify the meaning of intimacy or *love* in Sullivan's sense (wherein the satisfactions and security of the other person are as important to one as are one's own), we need to relate it to the social development of romantic love. Arnold Green (1952) with his usual perspicacity wrote:

> The function of "love" in modern society is peculiarly complex. In the past, personal relations tended to be rigidly defined and to involve entire personalities. With the decline of the traditional family, family relationships could no longer be held together with shared and integrated functions. The improvisation of total emotional involvement with others, or modern "love" in courtship, marriage, and family relations, appeared. When the old script which clearly outlined proper conduct was blurred, when the rights and obligations of husband and wife became more a matter to be settled by bargaining in each marriage, the answer of the culture was to jazz the tempo of *romantic love*.

This "love" is said to prepare its followers for a spiritualized idealization of the loved one which comes like a bolt out of the blue. In the twentieth century in the United States the idea that romance is to be *culminated* and *maintained* in marriage came to fruition. So powerful are prevailing cultural patterns in relation to "romantic love," that even though romantic love as an experience is purely cultural in origin and expression, adolescents—and many adults—fall in and out of love several times. People are "trained" to fall in love. And yet, as Green points out, it is the poorest possible basis for maintaining marriage. One reason is that such a notion of "love" is a highly stylized drama built around beauty and charm (Green, 1952). While there are other reasons which Green mentions, we shall abandon further discussion of the pitfalls of romantic love. However, it is important to mention that business enterprise has reaped billions of dollars by the exploitation of romance. From the early days of motion pictures to present day soap operas, this seems perfectly clear. Even when we buy a bar of soap, we are supposedly enhancing the opportunity for romantic fulfillment.

Psychologically speaking, Sullivan offers a much sounder framework of *intimacy* between two people, although it may seem to lack glamour. He characterized *intimacy* as that type of situation which permits validation of all components of personal worth. But what does validation mean in this context? Sullivan asserted that validation of personal worth requires a type of relationship which he called *collaboration*, that is, clearly formulated adjustments of one's behavior to the expressed needs of the other person in the pursuit of increasingly identical or more and more mutual satisfactions, and in the pursuit of security operations. Security operations are actions or stratagems to maintain, protect or enhance self-esteem.

The mutual validation of all components of personal worth by the chums is for the most part what Sullivan means by *love*. The start of *preadolescent intimacy* requires that certain factors be present such as "obvious likeness," parallel to physical development. Such factors are said to make for situations in which boys feel at ease with boys rather than girls. Thus, preadolescent intimacy presupposes a "feeling of species identity or identification" which influences the feeling involved in the preadolescent change. According to Sullivan, ordinarily, the capacity to love first involves a member of one's own sex (gender) — but is is not a sexual relationship. However, this does not deny the possibility that there are many people, as Sullivan believed, who do not progress psychologically beyond the juvenile era or regress from preadolescence to the juvenile era of *cooperation, competition* and *compromise*. When they reach adolescence or chronological adulthood, they may marry and support a family, but love is something they will never have to offer.

With the realization of preadolescence and the state of intimacy there follows in its wake a great increase in the *consensual validation* of symbols, of symbol operations, and of information, data about life and the world.

> This comes about as a fairly obvious consequence of the fact that the other fellow has now become highly significant to one. Whereas previously, one may have learned to say the right thing to one's companions, to do the right things, now these sayings and doings take on a very special significance. One's security is not imperiled by one's love object. One's satisfactions are facilitated by the love object. Therefore, naturally, for the first time one can begin to express oneself freely. If another person matters as much to you as do you yourself, it is quite possible to talk to this person as you have never talked to anyone before. The freedom which comes from this expanding of one's world of satisfaction and security to include two people, linked together by love, permits exchanges of nuances of meaning, permits investigations without fear of rebuff or humiliation, which greatly augments the consensual validation of all sorts of things, all of which in the end, symbols that stand for — refer to, represent — states of being in the world (Sullivan, 1953).

Sullivan claimed that as a result, one becomes more fully human in that he begins to appreciate the common humanity of people, that there comes a new sympathy for the other fellow, whether he be present to the senses, or known only through books and mass media. Learning now becomes a means of self-fulfillment, not a matter of pleasing teachers and parents. During preadolescence, the world expands as a "tissue of persons and interpersonal relations which are meaningful." Only then, Sullivan believed, does knowledge become truly significant, and learning becomes a serious attempt to implement oneself for one's future career.

Even in the case of those who are fortunate enough to enjoy an unalloyed preadolescence, one cannot safely predict a happy future. Sullivan wrote,

> I believe that for a great majority of our people preadolescence is the nearest that they come to untroubled human life—that from then on the stresses of life distort them to inferior caricatures of what they might have been (Sherif and Sherif, 1969).

PSYCHOTHERAPEUTIC POSSIBILITIES IN PREADOLESCENCE

The preadolescent phase of personality development frequently has very great inherent *psychotherapeutic possibilities*. It has been previously stated that the self-system is much more subject to change, either fortunate or unfortunate, at each of the developmental thresholds. Preadolescence has an "almost fantastically important" capacity for change in the self-system. Sullivan believed that in the Western world, a great deal of the activities of juveniles is along the lines of the ideals of an intensely competitive invidious society. Thus, competitiveness is built into our educational system—consider the struggle for good grades. Of course, it is possible that the other major aspects of the juvenile era, compromise and cooperation, may have gained in importance and influence during the past generation. Throughout the juvenile era, a youngster can have a very significantly distorted personification of the self while keeping it "under cover." This is a grave warp in the juvenile's personality. Since preadolescent intimacy provides an opportunity for correcting autistic, fantastic ideas about oneself and others, such a disturbed juvenile, if he is fortunate, may be able to become a close friend of another disturbed preadolescent. When this happens, the juvenile who reaches preadolescence, egocentric and handicapped, may experience an expansion of the self, and a more realistic appraisal of himself and others, with a new superior grasp of interpersonal relations, if he can learn to relate to some of his peers.

PREADOLESCENT SOCIETY

Sullivan claimed that there occurs in preadolescence the development "of at least an approach" to what sociologists of an earlier generation called "the gang." At present, the mention of the gang conjures up loose organizations of groups of males and females who are both individually and collectively antisocial. There are such gangs of course, but they are by no means synonymous with the essence of the gang as sociologists have described it or, for that matter, Sullivan. There are probably several factors which hinder the formation of the gang in the classic sociological sense. One factor may be the rapid population shifts in the large urban centers. Americans are notoriously "on the move." Some of the causes are racial, as in the case of Caucasians fleeing to the suburbs; others are socio-economic. The "mobility" of Americans since World War Two has been especially marked, apparently adding to the disruption of an older, more stable United States. In any case, the rate of social change seems to accelerate constantly so that families and neighborhoods in the larger cities seem to change in character overnight. Nevertheless, the tendency to form gangs remains. It seems to be almost ubiquitious as Sherif and Sherif (1969) point out. "The formation of small groups of buddies in the armed services is a well-documented fact, as it is in prisons, schools, neighborhoods, and social and business circles."

Yet, they identify the gang as applying only to youthful or adult groups that engage in socially undersirable or criminal behavior (Sherif and Sherif, 1969). Sullivan emphatically rejected this delimitation of the gang. He thought—probably correctly—that there is more literature on antisocial gangs than there is on the vastly favorable aspects of preadolescent society. He asserted,

> I believe that a study of preadolescent society in the very worst neighborhoods would reveal tendencies other than those leading toward becoming minor criminals. And in some very bad neighborhoods, while there are gangs which are antisocial, there are also gangs which are very much less antisocial, if not actually constituting a constructive element in the neighborhood (Sullivan, 1953).

Sullivan's suggestion came to fruition by O'Hagan's (1976) research project, carried out on such urban adolescent gangs from the west of Scotland. The results showed that in a large urban area different types of gangs may appear emphasizing differing aspects of group behavior. A continuum existed from a stable and organized gang to a transitory pole. Sullivan's notion of gang formation was proven to be farsignted by the finding that frequently gang members have no clear idea of how their gang originated or why it adopted a certain structure with an unwritten code of norms. It seems that no single theory can account for the many different characteristics of the juvenile and preadolescent gangs, although the socio-economic environment is of great importance.

The Male Preadolescent

Godpaille in his book *The Cycles of Sex* (1975) has written that between the ages of nine and twelve (the beginning of what Sullivan called preadolescence) the period of relative harmony between the child and his parents ends. He also claims that the youngster's body begins to prepare itself for sexual maturity through an even more sharply rising elaboration of sex hormones. This biochemical change is said not only to affect the child's body, but also his mind and emotions, and to set off a chain of personal and social responses that will not reach a state of equilibrium until the end of adolescence. In constrast, Sullivan would say that however important these biochemical occurrences may be, they only form a substrate to what he has in mind: "the quiet miracle of preadolescence." Normally, a new and complex level of interpersonal relations is reached which transcend the biochemical in a course of behavior. Passing references to the "social" and *its* effects are not enough. Life is lived—or simply endured on an interpersonal level. As long as that is clearly understood, we welcome Godpaille's formulations.

In order to sharpen his exposition, Godpaille (1973) characterized the specifically biological and anatomical series of changes which culminate in reproductive capacity. He wrote,

> Puberty is panhuman, and except for variations in timing and duration, in healthy humans everywhere it is an innate inexorable event that occurs at roughly the same time of life and with roughly the same sequence of maturational changes.

A girl is considered to have reached puberty at the time of menarche; a boy, when he is capable of ejaculation. Many investigators conceive adolescence as the psychological and socio-cultural response to puberty. Prepuberty designates the one or two years of accelerating biological changes that occur before the "arbitrary chosen peak" or midpoint marked by menarche or ejaculatory capacity. This period would be roughly characterized by Sullivan as preadolescence, or the beginning of preadolescence.

There are many changes leading to puberty, which cannot be discussed in detail owing to space limitations. It is thought that the onset of prepubertal changes is mediated by the hypothalamus. Puberty is said to be not merely an independent maturation of the primary and secondary sex organs, and other bodily parts. Their maturation is thought to be largely dependent upon hormones produced by the anterior pituitary gland which is controlled by the hypothalamus. (A detailed description of the relationships between the CNS and endocrine glands is unnecessary for the purposes of this book.)

> The essential role played by the hypothalamus, rather than by the level of maturation of the other organs involved, is demonstrated in one way by the fact that the premature circulation of gonadotropins—the pituitary hormones necessary for sexual maturation—will produce prococious puberty regardless of the child's age (Godpaille, 1975).

Thus puberty is said to be not merely an independent maturation of the primary and secondary sex organs.

The main male sex hormone, of many chemically similar androgens — testosterone — is responsible for essentially all the physical changes of male puberty. Godpaille has noted that biological and "intro psychic" circumstances combine to encourage a rejection and repression of the uncontrollable, the damaging and the feminine, in favor of the comforting repeatable pleasure and presence of the essential male organ, the penis.

A growing inner turmoil of preadolescents, according to Godpaille, has been emphasized, much more so than by Sullivan who conceived of preadolescence as constituting a new relationship to the world. Godpaille asserts the naturally increasing differences in the psychology and in the emotional task of boys and girls, and that it is a human characteristic to regress under stress when better dynamisms of adoptation are not available. But, for Sullivan, preadolescence is not naturally or usually an era when girls and boys regress to a time when the parents were splendid figures. (That is a Freudian idea which Sullivan would emphatically reject.) But we are aware that the mother plays a great role in the development of her daughter's self-identity and, if in turmoil, can more easily regress to the mother of infancy. But the boy's ego is said to be not fully prepared to cope with parental changes and regress to the "Oedipal phase" and so it may be that the boy tries to escape from his troubles by retreating into a gang. This explanation of gang formation strikes us as highly questionable. For Sullivan, it is a much more normal, if not a "natural" occurrence.

The Structure of Preadolescent Society

The preadolescent two-groups tend to interlock. Suppose that A and B are chums. It may happen that A also finds much that is admirable about C just as B finds much that is admirable about D. A linkage of interest may be formed among these two groups. But also C and E are chums as are D and F. And so the linkage of interest becomes extended. There is probably a limit to the number of two-groups who can form such a linkage but one can not specify it (Hare, 1955). Quite frequently, owing to his fortunate experience in earlier phases of development, there will be a particular outstanding preadolescent who serves as a model. As a result, he may become the third member of a number of two groups, such as those mentioned above. But like everyone in the preadolescent society, he may have a particular chum. The various two groups may be linked to this outstanding preadolescent as their leader and perhaps his particular chum as well. Basically, this forms the organization of the gang. Sullivan thought that the world is reflected in the "preadolescent microcosm."

Consequently, the gang as a whole has a relationship to the larger formal organization, the community which assesses the gang, and is likely to accept it or not depending on whether it is benign or antisocial. The gang's acceptance by the community may also depend on how widely representative of the community the gang is.

Types of Warp and Their Remedy

There are several types of warped juveniles who can be "put on the right road" toward a fairly adequate personality development once their need for intimacy has matured and they experience preadolescent socialization. First, it is important to mention *egocentric people* who go from childhood through the juvenile era and still retain literally unlimited expectations of attention and service to themselves. Some of them sulk when they do not receive attention. Under certain circumstances, some of them have temper tantrums. An egocentric juvenile may sometimes find a chum who is in somewhat the same position as himself during preadolescence. In such a case, each may do the other considerable good, gradually becoming less objectionable to the preadolescent society, so that eventually they may be esteemed by the gang. But not every egocentric juvenile will follow that route. Some two-groups made up of youngsters who have endured the ostracism of their peers may be so resentful that they seek out and identify themselves with the most antisocial leadership which can be found during preadolescence. Nevertheless, Sullivan held that even some of the juveniles who arrive at preadolescence strikingly marked with the malevolent transformation establish a chumship which in turn becomes integrated into the preadolescent gang, whereupon the malevolent transformation gradually disappears.

There is another type of person who believes that something is wrong with others if they don't like him. Such a person, while in the juvenile era, never learned that his attitude toward human life is not reasonable. He tries to handle his inevitable disappointments by rationalizations which belittle others and/or by disparagement of others, a very self-destructive stratagem for which he generally has experienced an excellent example of in his home. Despite such a handicap, some of these youths, when they get into preadolescent socialization, quite often gain enough in security from the new-found intimacy with their chums to open their minds. That is, for the first time in their lives they can discuss these other unpleasant people who don't like them with their chums in such a fashion that they gain insight into the real worth of the others as well as a measure of understanding of their own shortcomings. Thus, an exchange of views does not imply an immediate agreement, but rather a mutual exchange and comparing of notes. So, preadolescence is said to tend actually to correct, to a notable extent, one of the most vicious forms of morbidity widely prevalent among people in the United States, according to Sullivan, namely, the tendency to disparage and pull people down. Unfortunately, preadolescence cannot work miracles. But in many instances, it does tend to mitigate this all too easily acquired morbidity.

Still another type of warped youth is the one who "will not" grow up. In the juvenile era, he is sometimes popular though often he is unpopular. In any event he becomes increasingly unpopular as the juvenile era comes to its normal end. Sullivan claimed that this type of person can properly be called irresponsible. "He doesn't want to take on anything that he can avoid; he wants to remain, if you please, juvenile." Sullivan goes on to say that such a youth wants to be as young as possible, unwilling to bend the knee to society's necessities with respect to others. In some instances, such a youth benefits markedly from the maturation of the need for intimacy. In other instances, such a person gets into an irresponsible gang.

Sullivan sums up the various types of warp with the comment that as long as they do not preclude the formation of preadolescent intimacy which will provide for some checking and counterchecking of experience, that is, consensual validation, they are open to remedy. To the extent that a particular warp is remedied, the preadolescent's self system is definitely expanded, "and its more troublesome, inadequate, and inappropriate functions are reduced to the point that they become unnecessary" (Sullivan, 1953).

DISASTERS IN TIMING OF DEVELOPMENT STAGES

Since the beginnings and endings of the various eras are not fixed, the effect of previous experience on the rate of maturation becomes "peculiarly conspicuous" as the preadolescent progresses toward puberty. It is an established fact that the time of the puberty change may vary considerably from person to person. This seems to be caused not only by biological factors, but by experiential factors as well. Certain lamentable things can happen as a result.

A particular person may not have the need for intimacy at the statistically normal time. Therefore, as Sullivan puts it, "he does not have an opportunity of being part of the parade as it goes by." As the end of the parade begins to pass from sight, he may develop a need for intimacy, but now he is likely of necessity to establish a relationship with a chronologically younger person, since his contemporaries will have vanished into the vast scramble of adolescents for dates, parties, and what not. But a relationship with a younger person is not necessarily a great disaster. If the *delayed preadolescent* forms a relationship with an actually adolescent person he is more likely perhaps to begin a *modus vivendi* which ends as a homosexual way of life or at least a so-called bisexual way of life. Thus, he is forever cut off from the possiblilty of an intimate relationship with an adult member of the other sex — a relationship which is profoundly different in quality from the preadolescent chumship.

Sullivan claimed that the number of instances of schizophrenic disorder experienced by one of the chums — due to an arrest of development — while the others of his group, including his chums, have been progressing into adolescence, was in his experience, notable.

Loneliness

Loneliness has a developmental history. But, according to Sullivan, it reaches its full significance and intensity in the preadolescent era and goes on relatively unchanged throughout the rest of life. As an experience, loneliness is said to be so terrible and intimidating that it baffles clear recall. From infancy onward, various motivational systems or components appear stage by stage, which combine to form "quintessential loneliness" during preadolescence or at any time of life thereafter. This may change in quality. The first component appears in infancy as the need for contact, which in turn merges with the need for tenderness. But this need does not cease with the end of infancy, rather it extends into childhood, where additional components become evident as the need for adult participation in the child's activities. The need for compeers enters into the experience of loneliness during the juvenile era, so does the need for acceptance. Thus, in the juvenile era the fear of being accepted by *no one* of those whom one must have as models for learning — in other words, is a prelude to quintessential loneliness. Preadolescence, enhances the growth of the dreadful experience of loneliness by the addition of the need for an intimate exchange with a fellow human being, that is, the need for the most intimate type of exchange with respect to satisfactions and security.

There is a question about Sullivan's formulation of loneliness which over the years has been ignored. Sullivan knew that during adolescence, there is normally a shift in the intimacy need for a member of one's own sex to a member of the other sex. Yet, he never formuated it as an additional and ultimate component in the long evolution of loneliness. We do not interpret this as a sexual drive. No one has to be told — especially today — that (genital) heterosexual relations are thriving among the young people of the land, but it is highly questionable if there is much intimacy (in Sullivan's sense) involved in these affairs. Glamour and romance make such sexual activities more acceptable to many, although some young people eschew any such romantic tendencies and are openly exploitative. Biological differences, which in turn can scarcely be ignored in the psychological make-up of each sex, cultural differences due to the differently defined roles, unique experiences of each sex, the desire for children whether for biological or cultural or uniquely individual reasons—all these, in addition to lust, have always and everywhere throughout the civilized world, created a longing in normal people, who are not warped by current cultural trends, for intimacy with at least one member of the other sex. For such reasons, we conclude that Sullivan's admittedly brilliant formulation of loneliness is incomplete.

Loneliness is a more powerful driving force than anxiety and can compel people to seek companionship even though intensely anxious in the performance. Unhappily, people who seek companionship under such conditions, often show a serious defect of orientation in living, due to unfortunate past experience. The lack of necessary experiences and skills may make it impossible for a person to form a correct appraisal of the new situation in which he finds himself. And he becomes vulnerable to all sorts of misfortunes with his partner unless he is extraordinarily lucky—or hastens to some competent counseling service.

THE PREADOLESCENT FEMALE

Sullivan used to assert that he knew little about women. It wasn't true. Several women were in his "variant of psychoanalysis" with him. And many more were supervised or "controlled" their patients with him, still he was diffident or seemed to be when he "talked" about women.

Even so, he has not discussed the developmental sequence of girls. And so the following excerpt from Warren J. Godpaille may be very helpful in filling in this gap (Godpaille, 1975).

> We know, that there are characteristic differences between preadolescent boys and girls, in addition to their similarities. Girls are said often to appear to become even more emotionally disorganized. Apparently as a result of this disorganization, girls' attention span is often decreased and their ability to express themselves coherently sometimes seem totally lost. They endure mood swings that are more intense, more frequent, and more unpredictable. Their general sense of dissatisfaction with themselves and others are said to be at times seemingly overwhelming. As they approach menarche while their estrogen cycle becomes more regularly cyclic, coincidentally, as it were, so may their mood swings, though some premenstrual tension is unquestionably emotional in origin, not all of it is. The menses may not yet have begun, and progesterone may not be as prominent in prepubertal endocrinology as it will subsequently, so that a girl's mood swings may gradually assume a more regular timing (Sullivan, 1953).

Godpaille (1975) has asserted that this is not an inevitable development, but a perceptive observer may sometimes discern a faint preview in the rhythm of irritability, peacefulness, moodiness, enthusiasm, and depression.

Most of the ill temper of a preadolescent girl, expressed in transactions with her mother, often overtaxes the latter's patience and understanding. The father is said to be relatively exempt, and at times can be the only stabilizing influence in the home.

"Girls do not tend to form peer group gangs as boys do;" rather they form intense twosome friendships, often with overt sexual overtones, and are much given to sharing sexual secrets (Godpaille, 1975). Yet, these friendships often pursue a stormy course. During preadolescence, girls possess an "unparalleled advantage" for the expression of any malice which they may have been storing up. Girls possess a two-year lead in growth and sexual maturation. The female is not only taller and generally bigger, but is blossoming into young womanhood. Any reasons, real or fantasized, she may harbor for wanting to get back at boys can be now acted upon with relative impunity (Godpaille, 1975). During the preadolescent era, she can surpass a number of boys in sports and in school performances. Characteristic preadolescent feminine behavior is teasing boys.

One can see little in feminine dominance future harmony (Kestenberg, 1967). We know that boys subject to female dominance are woefully vulnerable. Normally, the first "object of identification" is a woman (mothering one)—whom someone has called the symbol of womanhood. Hence, boys are not as secure in their "sexual identity" (gender identity) as girls. The overbearing behavior of the latter "hits them" where their defenses are fragile and leaves them with little ability to fight back. Their tendency, as previously pointed out, is to band together in mutually reassuring all-boy gangs and make a great show of depreciating and repudiating girls and femaleness (Raz, 1971). Sullivan, on the other hand, thought that boys join to form gangs because this is an inevitable evolution in their social development. When prepubescent endocrine changes do begin to affect them, they are still two years behind, and the emotions and fantasies that are stirred and reawakened make them even more anxious about females and more defensively bonded together in their all-male group. The disjunction of male and female development is over stressed in contemporary life in the United States. One suspects that an element of "Women's Liberation" may have unconsciously influenced this trend. Another point is that the violence, hostility and crime so prevalent in the United States during recent years may have affected feminine development.

EARLY ADOLESCENCE

It is important to keep in mind that dating and courtship patterns vary greatly around the world. Sullivan's formulations of adolescence, apart from his discussion of puberty, apply in particular to the United States and Western Europe. In some parts of the world, cultural differences are so great, that the Sullivanian orientation simply would not apply. The beginning of *adolescence* which, as we saw in an earlier chapter, can be profoundly influenced by environmental factors, some of which may be physical, others cultural, is "ushered in" by the puberty change or what Sullivan called the "frank appearance of the genital lust dynamism." It may first be manifested by sexual orgasms in sleep, in the case of males, or in the occurrence of orgasm in play, which may occur if members of the gang, toward the end of preadolescence, engage in genital play or *auto-masturbation*.

Adolescence is differentiated into an early and late phase. *Early adolescence* is defined as a period of personality development from the eruption of true genital interest, lust, to the patterning of sexual behavior. The *patterning* of *sexual behavior* is the onset of *late adolescence*. There is a second characteristic of early adolescence, which is easy to expound theoretically, but, as Sullivan stated a generation ago, in actual fact leaves very much to be desired in the present-day American scene. This second characteristic is a change in the object of intimacy, from someone quite like oneself *(isophilic intimacy)* to the seeking of someone who is in a very significant sense (and possibly several significant senses) very different from oneself *(heterophilic intimacy)*. However, Sullivan held that certain cultural influences, such as the "double-standard," makes the shift in the intimacy need difficult.

But, even as Sullivan lectured, the "double standard" had begun to be undermined. Perhaps, one should take a backward look to the invention of Henry Ford's Model T. Cut loose from the influences of home, neighborhood, and church, young people by the millions have been bemused by romantic-love idealization. This is far from what Sullivan meant by heterophilic intimacy. Thus, a new pattern of man-woman behavior has appeared, as Arnold Green (1952) pointed out, there is among the young unmarried: "a long period of premarital dalliance, irresponsibility, and experimentation." There is, to this day, no evidence that this state of affairs has promoted and fostered love of man for woman or in Sullivan's terminology, heterophilic intimacy. Consider the divorce rate.

The change in choice of the "object" is said to be naturally influenced by the concomitant appearance of the genital drive. Why this is so, is not clear. But, the shift of interest toward the other sex in itself does not make intimacy difficult. In an indefinitely large proportion of the population it may foster it, although Sullivan does not say so.

Sullivan asserted that the new awakening of curiosity in the boy as to how he could get to be on as friendly terms with a girl as he has been with his chum is usually ushered in by a change of covert processes. His fantasies abruptly become altered from those of his preadolescent stage of development. As he reaches the terminal phase of preadolescence, his overt communicative processes may change in content. Individually and collectively, the chums may share whatever information they have picked up from older brothers, sisters, or friends. In this era of television, one doubts the value of most "shows." Frequently, they perpetuate the over-idealization of members of the opposite sex. However, many moving pictures portrayed in recent years deprive the female of her humanity and reduce her to an "object" or something to be exploited. Nevertheless, the romantic idealization of sexual behavior is still widely prevalent, despite the "new freedom" from traditional sexual mores.

Collisions of Lust, Security, and Intimacy Need

Traditionally, in the Western World *adolescence* has been a difficult period for many people. It is difficult to determine how much of the adolescent upheaval is caused by inhibition of the sexual (genital) drive. Do other problems which young people face become channeled into the tensions of the sexual drive? Once puberty is passed, one knows that the day when he can no longer rest secure in the parental home cannot be far off. Until fairly recently, graduation from high school marked the end of one's dependence on the home. At present, for great numbers of young people, graduation from college ends the relatively carefree period of life. One wonders what proportion of young people are in college in order to postpone the day when they will have to go out into the cold, indifferent, and impersonal world and seek work. One's parents cannot or will not support one indefinitely. As one ponders this situation, school days no longer seem so burdensome. For many registered students, who have little or no drive to broaden and deepen their education and who avoid the more difficult natural science courses on those late afternoons stretching from semester to semester, when they could congregate with like-minded fellows in some local beer parlor, in order to relieve the rigors of classroom lectures, quizzes, examinations, and professors who don't understand the problems of the new generation, those college years must seem happy ones indeed. If one's college has become co-ed, then both promise and opportunity have been magnified.

Apart from the small proportion of students who go on to graduate school, graduation puts an end to the halcyon days of freedom without responsibility. Therefore, it is necessary to distinguish the "problem" of adolescents who would avoid the responsibilities of adults from those who have been more seriously warped during the course of their personality development.

The first type of *conflict* which Sullivan mentions has perhaps less intensity than it did even one generation ago when many people regarded sex as disgusting and damned. He taught that the most ubiquitous collision is that which occurs between one's *lust* and one's *security*, that is, in this context, one's feeling of self-esteem and personal worth.

A generation ago, a great many people in early adolescence suffered much anxiety in connection with their "new-found" motivation for sexual (genital) activity. If one was brought up to believe that any sexual activity, apart from sexual intercourse within the bounds of matrimony, carried on for the sake of pleasure was wrong, then one was made very vulnerable. If one was in the company of a girl who made it evident that she expected some sort of sexual overture, what was one to do? Suppose she seemed to expect to be kissed. Then how does one go about kissing a girl if one does not know how? Especially, when one feels embarrassed, awkward and tense? In the movies, it was made to look very easy — once the great romantic overtures had been rehearsed. But what if one is a 15 or 16 year old boy, not a Clark Gable or a Paul Newman? The problem can be really a lot tougher than geometry or English composition.

But there is a far more difficult problem which, according to Sullivan, many people have suffered from, and which pertains to the genital area of the body, not necessarily related to any cultural peculiarity, although created from personal experience.

The rather profound problem, with respect to the genital area of the body, Sullivan called *primary genital phobia*. By this he meant an *enduring warp of personality*, often inculcated in late infancy and early childhood, which practically converts that area of the body into "something not quite of the body." In an earlier chapter, it was pointed out that certain mothers or mother surrogates, in order to restrict the exploratory functions of the hands, make "incredible efforts" to keep the young child from handling the genitals and the anus. When such anxious or upset mothers are successful, the relevant area of the body may become "distinctly related" to the "not-me" part of the personality. At adolescence, the youth who has undergone such an experience is virtually unable to arrive at any simple, conventional type of learning with regard to what he can do with the genital lust dynamism. If such a youth ever belonged to a gang, it will have disbanded, as its former members now are busy with dating, and partying whenever the opportunity presents itself. Hence, the wretchedly unfortunate youth who suffers primary genital phobia experiences loneliness, if nothing else, as it were, added to his misfortunes. Bedeviled by such burdens, his activities become comparatively pointless. Since he hears that his chronological peers are having delightful adventures with members of the oposite sex, while he is powerless to accomplish much of anything, he suffers humiliation and considerable loss of self-esteem.

The second outstanding form of conflict or "collision" is that between the shift in the intimacy need and the need for security when parents frown on the boy's or girl's efforts to relate to a member of the opposite sex. But, this conflict is likely to be enhanced by the fact that, in general, the social climate of the United States has been profoundly occupied with achievements which have not promoted either happiness or what used to be called the good life — the life of the mind or what "old fashioned" folk called the life of spirit.

Sullivan has alleged that two generic interests have absorbed the energies of Americans or, in the terminology of Charles de Gaulle, "Anglo-Saxons," even though for more than 100 years millions of them were of Irish or Italian extraction, to say nothing of Blacks and numerous ethnic and racial groups from Finland to China and Japan.

The other great interest pertains largely to the exploiting of incredibly rich natural resources, and the allied development of transportation and communication. In this gigantic task, Americans have succeeded perhaps far too well. But, we shall resist any discussion of the energy shortage which the natural scientists seem to think is, like sex, here to stay (at least for a long time). The essential point is that apart from a favored or lucky few who could become genuine aristocrats, Americans have, at least until recently, devoted their time and energy to the gigantic task of producing wealth from a great continent filled with vast resources. Sullivan (1956) said,

> Thus, the understanding of the essentials of life and the evolution of a culture which would include the development of charming ways of human intimacy have lagged. Americans have many erroneous prescriptions and few correct orientations for human intimacy and therefore are not apt to feel automatically secure — at the same time that they are impressed from all sides with the importance of the kind of paint they have on their houses and the number of horsepower in their cars.

Even though, according to Sullivan, Americans generally are a "not particularly friendly people," although they can be very genial, the need for intimacy (collaboration) reaches out toward and "settles on" a number of the opposite sex. Never mind, for the moment, that often intimacy with a member of either sex is all too brief, apparently because of the stresses of life. The striving normally exists, but there are numerous ways in which it can be thwarted, not by the particular girl (or boy, if the young adolescent is a female) but by certain elders in the home. Of course, such elders are perhaps a bit morbid, although there may be — one is not too sure — fewer than there were when Sullivan lived. At any rate, they bring "strong repressive influence" to bear on their offspring and they have at their disposal a potent instrument to which not only adolescents but most adults are vulnerable: ridicule. Ridicule is very hard on one's self-esteem, especially if he is a young adolescent. Whether the elders know it or not, ridicule is a very destructive weapon, for it tends to undermine the security of the boy (or girl) at a time when he needs as much self-assurance and self-confidence as he can possibly manage, especially since the member of the other sex he or she is reaching toward may not feel very secure, either. Such elders, usually parents, do not want their offspring to become interested in, as they interpret the situation, to get into trouble or dally with sex and all it could lead to, such as disease, marriage, and leaving home. Other elders, who are either too decent or ignorant of the destructive power of ridicule, interfere with, object to criticize, or employ some other technique which will hinder the early adolescent's efforts at achieving heterosexual intimacy.

A third type of conflict pertains to the *collisions between the* intimacy need and lust. Four varieties of awkwardnesses are said to be common, of which, three make up one group, namely, embarrassment, diffidences, and excessive precautions. These behavior patterns are familiar in one context or another so there seems to be no necessity to dwell on them. The fourth variety of awkwardness is called "the not technique," a stratagem designed to deny the existence of something by affirming its opposite, either in word or deed. Sullivan claimed that one of the ways of attempting to solve the collision between intimacy and lust is by adopting a stratagem which is the very opposite of diffidence, that is, a very bold approach in the pursuit of sexual (genital) satisfaction. Such an approach is so crude that it stamps upon the sensitivities and insecurities of the girl, making her embarrassed and diffident. Hence, the opportunity for the development of real intimacy is rendered quite improbable. This works both ways, so to speak. If it happens to be a girl who initiates behavior designed to satisfy *lust,* while employing the "not technique," she is likely to suffer the same fate. But traditional American cultural attitudes supposedly dictated that such sexual initiative originate with the male. It may be that changing definitions of woman's roles in life, combined with the invention of "the pill," have vastly reduced the probability of any of the four varieties of collisions.

In addition, increasingly there has been developing a notion that sexuality is more or less a commonplace affair and the source of great pleasure of which one should avail oneself at an early age, perhaps at the end of the Junior High School years, if not sooner. Apart from questions of morality, however important, other questions arise. How will intimacy fare in such relationships? Will they foster the growth of maturity? There are no unassailable answers to these questions and to related questions which have not been raised. It may be well to listen to what two well-known psychologists have to say about sexual behavior from a contemporary point of view.

It is expected that the next decade will see a manifold increase in our scientific knowledge about the nature of the sexual drive in human beings. It will also be interesting to observe whether "acceptable" sexual behavior will change the pervasive impact that sex motivation has on our behavior. Currently, sex sells not only itself (in the form of prostitution and pornography) but virtually anything it can be associated with, from girlie magazines and entertainment to automobiles, cigarettes, and even food . . . .

Will man become more hedonistic and dominated by sexual passion or less preoccupied and influenced by the lure of sex, as the "sexual revolution" of the seventies gains strength? (Ruch and Zimbardo, 1971)

If the reader is an undergraduate, perhaps temporarily isolated within the walls of some university, he may need to be reminded that the sexual revolution is only one of many kinds of revolutions occurring in the world: political, economic, social, etc. But, in 1980 it would be difficult to maintain such isolation. There is no room anymore for another Emily Dickinson.

LATE ADOLESCENCE

According to Sullivan, the distinction he made between early and late adolescence would not be needed in a social organization in which the culture provided the facilitation necessary for the patterning of sexual behavior. The "taboos" which he talked about have become loosened for a large proportion of the younger generation. As we have seen, it is not yet clearly known what the consequences of the sexual revolution will be.

Sullivan asserted that late adolescence extends from the patterning of preferred genital activity, through unnumbered educative and educive steps, to the establishment of a fully human or mature repertoire of interpersonal relations, as permitted by available opportunity, personal and cultural (Sullivan, 1953). There is a similar way of putting this, namely, that a person has reached late adolescence when he discovers what patterns of genital behavior he likes and how to fit them into the rest of his life. Of course, Sullivan's formula for late adolescence assumes several value judgments and should not be accepted uncritically. (This was also characteristic of Freud.) Sullivan's formula for late adolescence is not merely descriptive. It is normative or prescriptive, as well as descriptive. One of the influences which probably caused Sullivan to ignore many problems connected with sexuality, such as marriage and family life, is that he believed the failure to achieve late adolescence is the last blow, the crowning defeat for a great many warped, inadequately developed personalities. Whether this is as true in the 1980's as it was in the 1940's is debatable. But in any event, it does not resolve some of the problems related to one's *modus vivendi* in a given society. A sociologist, faced with the common problems which a society faces, such as fertility rates, population growth, marriage, family life, divorce, would be likely to look at what the individual likes and dislikes in a larger, broader context since the continued existence of the society is at stake.

One possible misunderstanding must be avoided. An adolescent's failure in his attempts at patterning his genital behavior, at fitting it into the rest of his life, is (or was) often such an all-absorbing, harrowing, frustrating experience — for no acts of will can avail against it — that it often constitutes the presenting difficulty which precedes the "erupting of very grave personality disorder" in an indefinitely large number of people. Nevertheless, Sullivan held that this kind of presenting difficulty is by no means the actual difficulty, the locus of which is always connected with the person's make up and his everyday relations with others.

The Importance of Opportunity

In discussing late adolescence, Sullivan tried to come to grips with some of the realities of socio-economic life. He stated that the outcome of late adolescence is so much a matter of accident that whether one continues to be, dynamically, a late adolescent throughout life, or actually someone that might reasonably be called humanly mature is often no particular reflection on anything more than one's socio-economic status and the like. Sullivan said opportunity is now a matter of other people and of gross social facilitation and prohibition. For example, until the famous "G.I. Bill" was passed after World War II, there were millions of youngsters who were too poor, or whose parents were too poor, for them to attend college. But, it has come about during the last generation that in a great many instances a Bachelor's degree does not take one very far on the road toward occupational success. In a great many instances, if one wants to enter the professions, he has to earn an advanced degree. But, even this is no guarantee of success in a highly competitive world. As for social facilitation, it often helps if one comes from a "good family," which usually means a family of some, perhaps considerable, affluence as well as social prestige. First of all, the chances are good that one has been reared in an environment where books and works of art are to some degree appreciated. Hence, unless one is stupid or unmotivated, learning is not so likely to be a problem. Second, it is more likely, once one has earned the necessary degrees, that family connections may sometimes open doors that are, or were until recently, closed to those who come from the "wrong side of the tracks."

To be sure, there are young people who reject "the Establishment" — at least temporarily. Contemporary writers have stressed a key problem which adolescents have presented to communities in the past decade, namely their challenge and flouting of authority (Gruggen and Pitt-Aikens, 1975). But, the contemporary industrial society leaves little room for high adventure. It is impossible to learn how many young men who rejected the usual opportunities have ended their brief adventure by getting a job as a park attendant or a taxi driver. Neither one of these jobs — and others one might name — fosters individuality and freedom. Of course, there is a much darker side to the problem of late adolescents, who despite educational opportunities, simply do not have the capacity to observe adequately and analyze the opportunities which are available. Sullivan once wrote that the average person, stripped of his illusory me-you patterns, would find himself surrounded by strangers. This lack of capacity may be due to inherent defect, various types of personality warp, or the more or less normal organization of the self.

It is important to mention that in Sullivan's life time the problem created by the "immigration" of Blacks from the South and the problems created by the immigration of Spanish speaking people had not yet surfaced, at least not noticeably. With regard to the problems of the Negro in the deep South, Sullivan was highly sympathetic (Sullivan, 1964). It may be more accurate to say that Sullivan was highly sympathetic to the problems of Negroes everywhere in the United States. But, the problems of Blacks and Spanish speaking people have now reached a different dimension. Racial and ethnic conflicts are becoming commonplace as the Negroes and Spanish speaking people struggle to obtain income, prestige, and deference. At present, this struggle has become national in scope. But it is chiefly the white middle classes who bear the brunt of the struggle, although not exclusively, since some of the new middle classes include the newer ethnic groups.

Growth of Experience in the Syntaxic Mode

If the "long stretch" of late adolescence is successful, or insofar as it is successful, there is a great development of experience in the syntaxic mode. Late adolescents who attend a university have extraordinary opportunity to learn, not only academic subjects, but the characteristics of people in a much broader perspective. The social sciences can provide a great deal of information about people in various parts of the world as well as some insights into their institutions. Unfortunately, a great many students have little interest in the past and thus have little interest in social science courses even though they can provide an enlightening perspective from which to view the present. But the long stretch of university life has more immediate importance. According to Sullivan, a university education gives the later adolescent an opportunity

> to observe his fellows . . . to discuss what has been presented and observed, to find out, on this basis, what in his past experience is inadequately grasped, and what is a natural springboard to grasping the new (Sullivan, 1953).

Sullivan believed that those who do not attend a university but instead become wage earners, "exploiters of their fellow man, or something or other," have more or less similar opportunities except for the lack of broad cultural interest that characterizes a good university. Almost anything one does in the process of earning a living provides opportunities to learn more about how to get on with people. The job provides opportunities to observe one's fellow workers, to exchange "views," to validate one's hunches.

Sullivan was a firm believer in the so-called work ethic. He said,

> In general, late adolescents are adults in the eyes of the law, and have all the benefits and handicaps thereunto appertaining. Thus they have to take on a good many responsibilities which are written into the culture . . . If they are fortunate, their growth goes on and on . . . (Sullivan, 1953)

INADEQUATE AND INAPPROPRIATE PERSONIFICATIONS OF THE SELF AND OTHERS

We normally think of ourselves and others as persons possessing reason, selfhood, and the like. The question to be raised is what sort of persons do we believe we are or others are. Do we think of ourselves as good or bad persons, wherein either the personification "good-me" or "bad-me" is predominant? Do we believe that other people, or most other people, when their life situations allow, are either "good" or "bad?" Or, do we adopt a more sophisticated attitude that people vary from those who are very good, according to conventional standards of the good, the mediocre (a mixture of good and bad traits), to the bad? In any event, one would have to fit such categories into a broad spectrum, always mindful of cultural differences and like. The fact that philosophers and psychologists have differed in their criteria of good and bad is not relevant in this context. The relevant problem is how do late adolescents experience themselves and others? That is the kind of problem that psychiatrists, for example, face daily, not only in regard to adolescents but to people who fall into a large number of different age groups. However, in the present context, we are concerned with late adolescents, though chronological adults are only superficially different, or even less mature, and may have regressed to the juvenille era.

Sullivan thought that a great many people don't seem to get very far along the long stretch of late adolescence, even though they have successfully negotiated the "sex problem," which itself, apart from personality warp, may not be any great problem in the 1980's. The mechanics of sexual behavior, for example, are usually not difficult. Moreover, these days there seems to be a plethora of young adults — who are willing to give an adolescent a helping hand, whether they are motivated by a desire for financial gain, pleasure, or the belief that sex is the royal road to high living. No, the problems connected with immaturity basically relate to anxiety, which, in turn, is an instrumentality of the self-system as it functions "within the personality," which, in turn, functions in the community.

At the level of consciousness, where communication is fairly easy, the critical opposition of anxiety is said to be manifest as people acquire views of themselves which are so far from valid formulations of their assets and liabilities, that these views are eternally "catching them" in situations in which the incongruity and inappropriateness of such situations are about to become evident to them, whereupon they suffer the interference of severe anxiety. Since anxiety interferes with alertness, with one's ability to analyze situations and therefore to learn from them, one does not see what he has contributed to many unfortunate and thwarting experiences. One does not get to understand himself very well. For personality, which includes the self, is made manifest in interpersonal situations only. The "intra-psychic" may be considered private, but chiefly in this sense it is the covert aspect of actions. Hunger, thirst, pain, love, hate, and pleasure have a subjective dimension. This is true to the point of triviality. But they mean little or nothing — even to the person who experiences them — until he has overtly manifested them and observed their consequences in actions — or observed other people's reactions to them. The fact that we possess memory and recall makes this point difficult for some to understand. Nevertheless, whether consciously or unwittingly, we are constantly drawing on past experiences in order to understand present situations, and in coming to grips with the novel.

Many late adolescents have gotten to be where they are with varying degrees of *warp* due to unfortunate past experiences. That is why they manifest superficially incomprehensible falsifications of their "views of themselves." They may believe they are "no good," "unlovable," "unattractive," "homosexual," or whatever. Unfortunately, their self-systems are usually resistant to change and learning from potentially educative situations. One may not say to such a person, "You are as good as the rest of us, but you always wear unattractive clothes, spend too much time cooped up in your room, fail to exercise initiative," etc. Such a person cannot believe what is true about himself in several areas of his living and might very well become extremely anxious if a well-meaning

acquaintance attempted to "show" him by the exercise of some
stratagem. It was Sullivan's belief that as you "judge" yourself, so shall
you judge others. Hence, the late adolescent who is bedeviled by a
warped self-system may not only lack much self-esteem, he will think
poorly of others as well. Any evidence which will contradict such "views"
may be evaded by the misuse of selective inattention.

Such a person may suffer numerous restrictions of living which are
attended by complex ways of getting at least partial satisfactions, and by
further complex processes "in the shape of sleep disorders and the like"
for discharging dangerous tensions. Sullivan said that these restrictions
of living, which lead to complex ways of getting only partial satisfaction,
and the accumulation of tension may be usefully considered from the
standpoint of "restricted contact with others and of restrictions of
interest." These restrictions cover a wide range; from the early
development of a shockingly isolated way of life, accompanied with such
great social distance that the late adolescent has to continue to deny
himself a great deal of useful educative and consensual validating
experience with others, to "circumscriptions" of oneself with the help of
such things as prejudice, caste, and class, if one happens to be in a very
small minority. One of the things Sullivan taught his students was never
to assume that the other person perceives or comprehends even the
seemingly most mundane "simple" situation in a fashion similar to
oneself. If it were feasible, similar advice might be given to a great many
young adults who have passed through a period of courtship and have
become "engaged," perhaps egged on by relatives who *mirabile dictu*, act
as though they believed every marriage is made in heaven. However,
such advice is virtually meaningless to a young couple who are soon to be
married. But time may serve as a harsh and costly substitute for the
advice of older, more experienced people.

Sullivan taught that there are also a great many instances in which the
restrictions of freedom of living are very much more striking in the sharp
circumscriptions of interest. In others, large numbers of aspects of living
are said to be, so to speak, taboo, for many people. A cumpulsory
restriction of living owing to unfortunate past experience may be masked
in the form of pseudo-social rituals and interests which superficially
appear to be quite different from a grave personal limitation. Sullivan
mentions devotion to games such as bridge. A generation ago, a very
select group of women of great socio-economic opportunities lived in New
York City. They did little each day but spend many hours—most of their
waking time—at a bridge club. They passed each day according to
Sullivan's ironic account, "with minimum talk to their husbands or
chauffeurs," and at the club they engaged in a highly ritualized
interchange with their fellows.

In more recent years, televison programs seem to serve as a substitute for living in the case of many people who, owing to personal warp, suffer grave restrictions of living. A great many of these programs are, of course, of interest only to those who are not discriminating, either in entertainment values or intellectual tastes. One has to be careful not to confuse people who suffer limitations of this sort because of personality warp with those who are confined owing to the dangers in a great many large cities of the United States.

Another type of restriction of living pertains to the development of ritual avoidances and ritual preoccupations. Sullivan chose an illustration from the realm of politics, where there seem to be ritualized avoidance in political matters. Since he lived through the era of New Deal legislation (in which he seems to have had a rather touching faith), he mentions avoidances that pertained to controversies which the New Deal aroused. Superficially, ritual avoidances and preoccupations may appear to be perhaps narrow specializations; but, they are not. The former entail the arousal of anxiety if one has any interest in a particular field. For example, the entire field of Marxist thought seems to be closed off to a very large number of students. If an instructor urges a class of students to study something of the philosophy (or ideology) upon which Russian communism is based, namely, Marxism-Leninism, one frequently meets with a tense silence or a vacuous stare. The argument that one should know the "philosophy" of one's country's powerful political adversary as a rule meets with no success. But an argument for the importance of studying Conservative thought would meet with similar failure. Finally, our imaginary instructor would probably discover that most people avoid philosophy in its entirety — except for a rare few who, for one reason or another, develop an interest in this highly abstract — but not necessarily "irrelevant" — field of thought. Of course, some people lack ability for work in any field of abstract thought and others are bored with anything that does not seem "practical." Even so, a university that attempts to educate students, confronts them at every turn with materials bearing on philosophical subject matter even if it is sometimes presented in a somewhat "popular," watered down version.

For students who are made anxious by a given subject matter or area of study, there is ready at hand a tradition going back at least two or three generations in American universities, which labels a course of study that is taboo as offering nothing more than "crap courses." Majors in the natural sciences and engineering, who are uniformly very bright, are often prone to avoid the entire field of the arts. Whether because of lack of imagination or some peculiar warp which makes the relatively straightforward forumlae and the ingenious techniques of the natural sciences on the undergraduate level peculiarly attractive, a great many bright and gifted students have managed to avoid any appreciation of what are perhaps man's greatest achievements. And this has occurred despite the efforts of various school officials who set up minimum requirements in the field of art studies. A bright science major can even "take" arts courses and pass them without the faintest notion of what he has been exposed to. He can memorize the characters and scenes of a play, learn the "story," take careful class notes and still learn nothing though he passes the course. There is no way to measure the peculiar understanding and appreciation required of a student of Macbeth or Tennyson's poetry, or the history of art. So, a bright physics major may pass a course in the arts with ease and still lack any appreciation of the plays or novels to which he was exposed.

On the other hand, arts majors often manifest disdain for the natural sciences. Some of them may say they are "no good" at science. They fail to see the beauty of the logic of the natural sciences and they are clumsy in the lab. And so many arts majors avoid science courses because it appears these courses make them feel insecure.

Summarily, it appears that an indefinitely large number of very bright or talented students are psychologically unable to learn much, if anything, of a given area of study because they do not feel secure with it. This does not seem to be due to lack of capacity or lack of fundamental interest, but some personal inadequacy. They avoid or evade it as best they can, employ verbalisms to denigrate it, and fall back on various rituals or rigid patterns of thought and behavior reminiscent of obsessive-compulsive pathology in order to protect their security.

SELF-RESPECT AND HUMAN MATURITY

Certain sections of *The Psychiatric Interview* (Sullivan, 1954), give a better idea of Sullivan's ideas on human maturity than any of his other lecture series. The psychiatric interview will be outlined in the last chapter of this book. Some things, however, are clearly stated. The mature person is one who has self-respect and respect for others. This is a necessary condition of maturity. It entails a realistic self-confidence. To a large degree, it involves freedom from warp, from severe vulnerability to anxiety, and the like. Sullivan surmised that each of the outstanding achievements of the developmental eras will be outstandingly manifest in the mature personality—for example, intimacy with the one other person and preferably more than one. By "eternally widening interests or by deepening interests or both" life continues to grow in significance. The world becomes of continually greater interest. Hence, it is not apt to become boring.

Sullivan asserted that psychiatrists have little professional contact with mature persons for the very good reaon that the latter do not need their help.

One should bear in mind that maturity is never an "absolute." It is limited by time and circumstances, personal and social. Psychologists and psychiatrists often equate maturity with *adaptation* or "adjustment." This sort of criterion has many merits, since we are in eternal transaction with the environment at all levels, directly or indirectly. Even so, one has to be cautious. The contemporary world is in such a rapid flux that a young person is becoming more and more in danger of embarking on a vast sea in a rudderless ship with no compass to guide him as he sets forth on life's journey. Many of the values of the contemporary social milieu in the United States or elsewhere may turn out to be chimerical. Perhaps because of its wealth, the United States seems to be a peculiarly fertile ground for false prophets: religious, moral, political, social, etc. As Allport might say, the great thinkers of the past from antiquity onward may serve as the best guides in the search for mature, rational human values. But, one should bear Spinoza's dictum in mind: "All things noble are as difficult as they are rare."

REFERENCES

Beach, F.A. ed. *Human Sexuality in Four Perspectives.* Johns Hopkins Press, Baltimore, 1977.

Godpaille, W. *The Cycle of Sex.* Charles Scribner's Sons, New York, 1975.

Green, A.W. *Sociology.* McGraw-Hill, New York, 1952.

Gruggen, P., and Pitt-Aikens, T. Authority as key factor in adolescent disturbance. *Brit. J. Med. Psychol.* 1975; 48: 153–159.

Hare, P. Borgatta, E.F., and Bales, R.F. eds.. *Small Groups.* Alfred A. Knopf, New York, 1955.

Kestenberg, J.S. Phases of adolescence — with suggestions for a correction of psychic and hormonal organizations. Part II — Prepuberty diffusion and reintegration. *J. Am. Acad. Child Psychiat.* 1967; 6: 577.

O'Hagan, F.J. Gang characteristics: Empirical survey. *J. Child Psych. Psychiat.* 1976; 17: 304–314.

Raz, R.K. *The Child From 9 —13: The Psychology of Preadolescence and Early Puberty.* Aldine, Chicago, 1971.

Rosenblith, J.F. and Allinsmith, W. *The Causes of Behavior: Readings in Child Development and Educational Psychology.* Allyn and Bacon, Boston, 1966.

Ruch, F.L. and Zimbardo, P.G. *Psychology and Life.* 8th ed.. Scott, Foresman, Glenview, Ill., 1971.

Sherif, M. and Sherif, C.W. *Social Psychology.* Harper and Row, New York, 1969.

Sullivan, H.S. *Conceptions of Modern Psychiatry.* W.W. Norton, New York, 1953.

Sullivan, H.S. *The Interpersonal Theory of Psychiatry.* W.W. Norton, New York, 1953.

Sullivan, H.S. *The Psychiatric Interview.* W.W. Norton, New York, 1954.

Sullivan, H.S. *Clinical Studies in Psychiatry.* W.W. Norton, New York, 1956.

Sullivan, H.S. *The Fusion of Psychiatry and Social Science.* W.W. Norton, New York, 1964.

6

Dynamisms of Difficult Mental Disorders

This chapter begins with the simplest definition of personality to be found in Sullivan's writings and lectures. Personality *"is the relatively enduring pattern of recurrent interpersonal situations which characterize a human life"* (Sullivan, 1953). The organism's relatively enduring pattern of recurrent interpersonal relations is what, in the main, characterizes a person. In the later years of his professional life, Sullivan got very defensive about the uniqueness of any person. Perhaps he was reacting against an excessive emphasis on individuality. One is dealing with different levels of reality. Hence, it seems wise to ignore this highly technical and controversial topic.

For the sake of expounding his ideas, Sullivan generally talked as if the self did this and that, just as other psychiatrists have written that the ego performed numerous functions of various kinds. This sort of stratagem has to be understood for what it is — a device which helps one's exposition along a difficult and winding road. It is always the person who thinks, feels, and acts. But, his being in the world governs all his experiences and behavior. In other words, when the person thinks, feels and acts he is engaging in a transaction.

Returning to a previous formulation, one cannot walk without a ground to walk upon. Analogously, one cannot think without the language and culture which exist in his community and which he has acquired, although thinking is by no means synonymous with verbal behavior. Of course, one can arbitrarily rule out, omit, the "inner" or subjective side of all human actions. Perhaps, for some purposes, that is perfectly all right. But it is not all right for most clinicians. The behavioral frame of reference is necessary — but it is not sufficient. There is no evidence known that the "inner life," the subjective or "mental" aspect of overt behavior is inefficacious. The fact that it is not amenable to the techniques of physics constitutes no logical argument for its abandonment. Pavlov, Watson, and others were dogmatists. Yet, we are told that dogmatism has no place in science. It seems very unlikely that the genial and gifted John B. Watson ever experienced an anxiety attack. An anxiety attack, however, can be very educative. Professor Watson might, if he had had such an experience, have been more respectful of the mental thought. It took a great deal to deflect Professor Watson from his appointed task.

In any case, the individual "possesses" a self—in Sullivan's sense. But every person, to some degree, has another side to his make up. Sullivan called it the *dissociated*. Normally, the person does not know anything about it—and definitely does not want to know anything about it. If one attempts to talk about it with him, one will in all likelihood meet with a blank stare and earn a reputation for being "weird." The cause of his ignorance and "resistance" is not difficult to fathom. It tends to arouse anxiety, which seems to be so pervasive that it has become almost a cliché in certain circles. In any event, anxiety is never welcome—no one wants it. In everyday life, perhaps only "quintessential loneliness" is more dreadful. Hence, a great many people engage in the unwitting misuse of selective inattention in order to evade or minimize threats to one's self-esteem. Those who are considered mentally disordered are compelled to employ not only selective inattention but an indefinitely large number of other stratagems or security operations in the attempt to ward off anxiety. Even the person considered normal by most standards is not always so secure that he can forever discard the various stratagems to protect self-esteem.

THE MEANING OF THE DEVELOPMENTAL APPROACH

Sullivan stated "a great many phenomena in the whole biological field are easier to understand if you trace them from their beginnings to their most complex manifestations." In Chapter One of *The Interpersonal Theory of Psychiatry*, Sullivan (1953) tries to explain why he believes this is so. In the same chapter, he also said that if one goes with almost microscopic care over how anybody comes to be what he is at chronologic adulthood, then perhaps one can learn a good deal of what is highly probable about living and difficulties in living. For example,

> Before speech is learned, every human being, even those in the lower imbecile class, has learned certain gross patterns of relationship with a parent, or with someone who mothers him. Those gross patterns become the utterly buried but quite firm foundations on which a great deal more is superimposed or built (Sullivan, 1953).

And the only way that occurred to him of communicating his "views" on these and related matters was by a careful "following" of that which is possible and probable from birth onward. (Compare John Herman Randall Jr., 1958.)

The developmental approach is quite clearly radically different from the organicist approach. The reader may know that the neuroses (a badly misused term) are usually classed as functional and so are certain psychoses, such as schizophrenia, for example, while other psychoses are said to be unquestionably "organic." For example, many people, either because of disease or physical injury, have suffered grave impairment of the central nervous system.

Sullivan was well aware of the organic etiologies in certain mental disorders although it was not a major field of interest for him. It was the functional mental disorders that he was primarily concerned with. Sullivan was aware of the difficulties that the clinician may face in distinguishing between organic and functional disorders. Organic Mental Syndromes such as, delirium, intoxication states, withdrawal states, and dementia can produce irreversible damage to the central nervous system and reduce a person to a "mindless like" organism or even kill him. There is other literature in which this subject is dealt with thoroughly, such as, the Diagnostic and Statistical Manual of Mental Disorders (1980) prepared by the Task Force on Nomenclature and Statistics of the American Psychiatric Association or *The Harvard Guide to Modern Psychiatry*.

Sullivan was a functionalist, or rather a genetic-functionalist. That is, he believed that one must try to understand and "treat" people who suffer difficulties in living because of their particular (unfortunate, sometimes disastrous) career-line beginning perhaps in infancy. This approach was not original with Sullivan as Havens in his masterly book *Approaches to the Mind* (Havens, 1973) has demonstrated. The following summarizes Sullivan's point of view:

> Now the syndromes which are most useful in the diagnosis of personal situations, come more and more clearly to appear to be statements of the past, the momentary present, and the future of the career of the person who is our subject. The career that we are discussing is made up of the events which have connected, now connect, and will presently connect him with the lives of other persons (Sullivan, 1953).

Mental disorders or difficulties in living are processes, Sullivan said, which, although they are a part of every personality, are at the same time the particular parts of the personal equipment that are often misused. These dynamisms which cause difficulty go into operation in interpersonal situations that do not achieve a goal, or that at best achieve only an unsatisfactory goal. Their frequent recurrence or their tendency to occupy long stretches of time is said to characterize the mentally sick as distinguished from the comparatively well.

It is important to emphasize that the functional significance of a particular dynamism characterizing a given mental disorder, namely, a concurrence of signs and symptoms frequently encountered by the therapist, the abstracting of which form the flux of events, is presumed to be based on a valid insight into human life.

> It is the extraordinary dependence of a personality on a particular dynamism that is, I suppose, the fundamental conception to have in mind in thinking of mental disorder. The schizophrenic patient, for instance, is often a person who has in the past persistently shown the dynamism which we call dissociation as a means of resolving the conflict between powerful needs and the restrictions which the self imposes upon the satisfaction of these needs. That is, people who have dissociated anything as powerful as lust, for example, are in great danger of schizophrenic collapse (Sullivan, 1953).

Since perhaps everyone manifests at least temporary troublesome difficulties in living, Sullivan concentrated his energies and efforts on certain major patterns of difficulties — "the so-called clinical entities" — and particularly schizophrenia and "obsessionalism" as it is manifested chiefly in obsessive-compulsive neuroses. But he has valuable ideas on various other clinical entities, some of which will be discussed in this and the next chapter.

HYPOCHONDRIA

Sullivan's approach to mental disorder is revealed, elegantly, in the following passage:

> If one cuts oneself off so completely from intimacies with others that, at the level of verbal communication, the only dependable topic is the wretched state of one's health, as in hypochondria, one is very much more shut out from a moderately satisfactory life than if one restricts these communicative and cognitive aspects to how wretchedly one is being abused by other people — by particular, specific other people — as in the paranoid state. The cost of maintaining a self-system in which the sentient flux from the interior of the body is the only matter that can be attended to *in extenso* is that most of the personality must be reduced to a much earlier state (Sullivan, 1956).

Sullivan did not spend much time enumerating symptoms, physical or otherwise. Nevertheless, the hypochondriac feels compelled to tell the therapist about them. His illness has become the presenting aspect of his personality. But, he is not preying on sympathy. He must discuss his illness even to someone who is delighted to hear of his suffering. The physical ailment is said to be a means for augmenting the person's security. "Without it, the patient would feel abased, inferior, and without any merit for the consideration of others" (Sullivan, 1953). Sullivan goes on to say that it is as if the source of chronic unworthiness which is obliterated as a subject of the person's consciousness by the obsessional routine is handled in hypochondriacal people on the level of obsession with the somatic symptoms and thinking about them.

Young physicians or young therapists sometimes become so impressed with the hypochondriac's symptoms that they attempt to treat them or refer the patient to someone who presumably will. In his typical ironic fashion—an attitude which puzzles or irritates some therapists— Sullivan relates that the hypochondriac is busily engaged in counting up his heart ticks, "or something of that kind," and telling the physician all about it, sometimes with every sign of being able to keep on indefinitely on the subject. But he is not enjoying himself. His lust "is gummed up; all sorts of things are gummed up." Often, his appetite is too. So, he is not enjoying many satisfactions. Even the experience of hunger and the satisfaction of food "is all gone by the board unutterably." The "integrative tendencies" or drives for satisfaction have reverted to, or regressed to, a much earlier level of satisfaction. Since regression is a very important explanatory concept, it is important to be clear about it, however troublesome it may be theoretically. Sullivan says,

> Take, for example, lust. If the lust dynamism regresses (reverts) below the level of preadolescence . . . the person would be engaging in prurient stories and obscene jokes, peering into the neighbor's windows at night, and all that sort of thing. Regression still further back we see only, I think, in the genito-urinary hypochondriac, and there it is very closely related to schizophrenia. The symptoms show, in some cases, the same degree of regression that we see in certain of the schizophrenic masturbatory activites—namely, regression to the point of reactivation of urethral components of the orgasm, and so on. They have experiences with a drop of mucus, for instance, in lieu of anything which ultimately becomes the genital dynamism (Sullivan, 1956).

But, the regression of the hypochondriac is by no means confined to the drives for satisfaction. The cognitive aspects of his personality are also "gummed up" so that at times his speech becomes autistic. Apart from certain feelings (affects), such as a pleasant interest in his illness, he seems to experience little of the positive emotions which life brings. His regression to earlier types of functional activity seems relatively comprehensive.

The source of the hypochondriac's problem is in the structure of the self dynamism, which is marked by a prevailingly negative attitude toward himself and others. By engaging others in a discussion of his malady, he is striving to overcome his felt unworthiness by a magical power over them. (No connections between means and ends.) Without the physical ailment, he would feel abased, inferior, and without any merit for consideration by others. Even though he manifests intense anxiety, it is always anxiety about impending physical doom—not about interpersonal situations. In this fashion, what Sullivan called the hypochondriacal dynamism in a way actually blunts the "utility" or efficacy of anxiety.

Due to the fact that the satisfactions of the hypochondriac have become truncated and his security fragile, he does not live in the same sense other people do—except perhaps when he is telling someone about his symptoms. That seems to be his chief way of relating to life—such as it is. Nevertheless, he cannot withdraw from the world of people, like the hebephrenic (disorganized type of schizophrenic disorder acccording to DSM III nosology).

ALGOLAGNIA

According to Sullivan, in algolagnia, it is the world, rather than the body that is regarded as ailing. "Algolagnics," he says, "are possibly the most gifted of all people at taking the joy out of life." They "suffer life"—and seem to enjoy passing their suffering to others. Owing to their particular warp, only life's unpleasant aspects seem to interest them. Hence, it is very difficult to lead them to manifest any interest in anything that is hopeful or pleasant. Their astigmatic slant on life is well illustrated by the following brief description.

> One of them, on his first trip abroad, rode on the "Coronation Scot" from Glasgow to London. He read a detective story throughout the journey, only thrice glancing out of the window. Finding himself observed, he remarked to his companion "Isn't the landscape boring." Asking as to the book in which he had seemed to be absorbed, he said that it was very tiresome (Sullivan, 1953).

He continued in this vein, mentioning in retrospect that the English trains were bad, the food tasteless and the money beyond his comprehension. (This episode occurred before World War II.) Apparently, everything he noticed was bad, wrong, or positively distressing. "A grim possibility could be found behind any piece of good news; a high probability of evil lurked in every promise." Sullivan described this person as an artist of great talent who did practically no work because he was so distracted with suffering caused by him by life, including the suffering of his family.

Like the hypochondriac, the algolagnic has to have a hearer—someone to serve as an audience. Moreover, sometimes the algolagnic and the hypochondriacal states overlap. That is, people who are exclusively concerned with their ill health may, on occasion, shift their concern to the disastrous state of the world. Sullivan asserted that the algolagnics are apt to be very much more intact than the hypochondriacs in the sense of having preserved their relatively contemporary motivational systems. That is a way of saying the algolagnics are not compelled by their particular warp to regress to any great extent. But, they nevertheless are immature personalities. Sullivan thought that algolagnia is a distortion which begins in the juvenile era or at least certainly appears in preadolescence, and represents an inadequate fruition of preadolescent development. His "sex life" is probably confined to the autogenital, though he may use a sex partner as an instrumentality instead of his own hands.

As previously noted, there is not a particularly conspicuous element of regression in a person whose adaptation to life is algolagnic. The algolagnic process is said to be more a way of handling a good deal of hatred (fear and anger), and, as such, appears to reflect what can happen to a person who has been subjected to extremely deleterious influences from a certain point in comparatively early life. Although the person who undergoes the algolagnic process must have experienced some affection and security in the beginning, he got bogged down — suffered an arrest of development — fairly early in life. By recounting how wretchedly he is being treated by the world, he discovered he could put others at a disadvantage. In so far as he can make others discomposed and embarrassed, they will serve his purpose. If he can "milk" not only sympathy, but money or something else of a similar nature from other people, then he has a seemingly very effective security device.

Algolagnia is a term that was coined by Schrenck Notzing in 1899 to cover both sadism and masochism. Sullivan used this term to describe a specific clinical syndrome.

In today's updated Nosology of Mental Disorders (see DSM III, 1980) the term Algolagnia is not used. But, from clinical experience, one knows that the patients described by Sullivan as suffering from this condition to exist and do not meet fully the criteria for the diagnosis of any mental disorder classified in the updated DSM III. We believe that is an oversight that should be corrected.

THE PARANOID CONDITION

While Sullivan's ideas will be expounded upon at length in the next chapter on the paranoid dynamism, an introductory survey in this chapter will help make the complexities of schizophrenia in the next chapter more intelligible. In *Conceptions of Modern Psychiatry*, Sullivan

(1953) claimed that the paranoid, the algolagnic, the hypochondriacal, and the obsessional states are probably different patterns of much the same maladjustive process. But in *Clinical Studies in Psychiatry*, (Sullivan, 1956), which represents a later stage in Sullivan's thinking, he seems to have modified this idea. According to the later formulation, hypochondria, algolagnia, and paranoia are discussed without reference to obsessionalism which is outlined independently. In any case, his views on the obsessional personality can be more conveniently outlined toward the end of this chapter, since he thought there is a distinct connection between obsessionalism and schizophrenia.

> The so-called paranoid condition requires the algolagnic, you might say, as a spring-board; but nonetheless it has a close connection with the hypochondriacal, if for no other reason than that it can clinically alternate with the hypochondriacal state (Sullivan, 1956).

Pure paranoia, Sullivan goes on to say, is one imaginary pole and pure schizophrenia the other. Paranoid individuals regard themselves as the victims of specific, deliberate injury by other people. In other words, they regard themselves as persecuted. The only durable relationships which they sustain are those in which they believe the other person is doing them an injury. Sullivan claims that if they are seriously disordered, the others in their interpersonal relations tend to be highly illusory. If they become interested in someone, the latter is "soon discovered" to be an agent of some persecuting agency, even if sometimes an involuntary one.

"The single most illuminating thing that I know about the paranoid condition," Sullivan (1956) asserted, "is its alternation with the hypochondriacal state." Although the alternation is not frequent, it does occur. Apparently, Sullivan saw patients who at one stage or period of the interview were hypochondriacal. Then, at some indefinite point they became paranoid, in the sense that they manifested paranoid ideas typical of the paranoid state. This development coincided with a marked improvement in their physical health. On the other hand, if their health began to deteriorate, paranoid ideas started to disappear.

Sullivan (1956) asserts that the central question in the two conditions (hypochondria and paranoia) is: what "becomes of the needs for satisfaction?" He goes on to say that the paranoid dynamism works beautifully in achieving security (at least relatively) for how can one avoid respecting oneself, the very embodiment of goodness, if one has been persecuted and driven by surrounding enemies into a state of impotence? The paranoid transference of blame can work marvels to protect one's conscious feeling of personal worth. Yet it has a built-in flaw that can be near fatal. Everyone must exist as a social being, "in interpersonal relations," or deteriorate. And, if other people, perhaps some of whom one tends to be attached, are persecuting him, then they cannot be sources of satisfaction. Nor can one sort out some of those others and exclude them as objects of blame because they are potential sources of satisfaction. The cause of that state of affairs lies in the way everyone is brought up. The very people who are the original sources of one's satisfactions were the same people who "conditioned" him to need security and in the process reinforced the twin-headed drives for satisfaction and security. Hence, all through life, the person's emotional and motivational sets tend to be as inseparable as the leaves of a shamrock or the roots from the trunk of a tree. One wants satisfaction from the same people from whom one wants security — and they are the ones to whom one is drawn close enough that they can wound by criticism, diminish one's self-esteem in numerous ways by word or deed, and, it may be, become a menace to one's security. As a result "the paranoid solution" makes it very difficult to be in a constructive integration, a positive relationship with another person who can provide satisfaction of one kind or another, as well as esteem.

Like the hypochondriac's, the "paranoid's" needs for satisfaction have to undergo regressive distortion of activities of an earlier level of development. Nevertheless, at times, a person suffering the paranoid condition so severely that he is psychotic may manage to get out of the hospital and have a sexual relationship with a member of the opposite sex. Investigation reveals, however, that there is a great social gap between the very temporary sexual partners. From a paranoid male's point of view, the female with whom he is having an "affair" is scarcely a human being. She is said to be more "a fantasy product" of this than a person who can be critical, threatening, or simply a human being with the usual complement of positive and negative characteristics. This kind of behavior is carried on with the help of a large amount of autistic (parataxic) fantasy.

The person who "transfers" all his faults to another in order to preserve at least a measure of security cannot maintain a relationship for long with anyone who was once significant to him and, therefore, dangerous because the latter might point out his intolerable weaknesses. So, the paranoid cannot completely "disfigure" reality. Sullivan's comments on the self in relation to the transference of blame dynamism is very illuminating. He said:

> The self-system is always a device for maintaining security with our fellows and for keeping intact the illusions of them that make up our mores, social prescriptions, and so on. Thus in the paranoid, the self-system continues to function to entangle into the protective system anybody who would be critical or with whom one would be exposed to criticism. It faces society in general hostilely and with danger flags flying from all parapets. It permits

relationships which are sometimes pretty fantastic, but still may be quite physically intimate and sometimes of reasonably considerable ("considerate," according to the text) intimacy, but only with people who do not present much danger in the sense of reminding the person of what really ails him (Sullivan, 1956).

HYSTERIA

Havens (1973) has written:

William Osler said, "Know syphilis and you know all of medicine." Know hysteria or schizophrenia and you come round, more or less the worse for wear, to most of the critical observations and fundamental disagreements in psychopathology.

There is a brief, non-technical, and lucid account of hysteria (conversion reaction) by John C. Nemiah in the *Comprehensive Textbook of Psychiatry* (1980). And a chapter by the same author in *The Harvard Guide to Modern Psychiatry*. Some of Pierre Janet's ideas are expounded by Havens in his *Approaches to the Mind* (1973) in a brilliant fashion. After quoting an excerpt from one of Janet's case histories, concerning a young girl 20 years old whose despair, caused by her mother's death, has made her ill, Havens (1973) has written:

Attention (by Janet) is called to the heightening of function. She remembered and repeated every detail. She appeared not merely to imagine the original scene but to hallucinate it. Another patient, in walking life paralyzed from the waist down, at night nimbly climbed among rooftops. Memory, imagination, motor skills were sharpened and inspired. We are asked to notice also the variety of ways in which the traumatic scenes returned. In one attack she observed, in another, participated. Still another vomiting, or a lump in the throat. These last, Janet suggested, represent the same memories and ideas as the somnambulisms. Ideas, pale creatures for the rest of us, are carried up into hallucinations, fits, changes in feeling and movement.

Despite Janet's great ability, he did not, according to Havens, and others, have Charcot's or Freud's relentless curiosity. He did not possess

their eagerness to throw caution, order, and convention to the winds and follow the surprising, scandalous, and unexpected. Much that mental patients did and felt disgusted him; he called them weak, degraded, lazy (Havens, 1973).

However, in his interpretation of schizophrenia, Sullivan borrowed certain ideas of Janet, such as coconsciousness, "separate, organized centers of attention, receiving impressions and able to be communicated with, in control of the personality..."(Havens, 1973). Sullivan used the same conception to understand and treat the schizophrenic ego. However, Sullivan was not in the least repelled by the bizarre behaviors of schizophrenics. And he was well aware of the role of conflict, unlike Janet.

Coconsciousness and unconsciousness are not different names for the same thing, although they are both formulations of dissociated states, that is, aspects of the personality which have been "split" from the control of consciousness or the "ego." An exposition of dissociation is too technical for a book like this one. William James in his *Principles of Psychology* (1880) has expounded the origins of *dissociation*, which can be traced to Charcot, Janet and Freud.

Havens (1973), with his usual lucidity, makes these distinctions clear. He wrote: "It was obvious to both Janet and Freud that the conscious ideas of the patient did not encompass the phenomena of hysteria. Freud then searched, first by hypnosis and later by the method of free associations, for *unconscious* ideas and was led forward to the idea of unconscious yearnings, attitudes, convictions, and expectations. Janet searched for what *besides* ideas was dissociated, and in what ways. He left behind the old conception of single ideas, resulting from trauma and splitting off from mental life, for that of dissociated functions or systems within which many sensations, acts, fears, and ideas were included.

> Hysteria was therefore the ideas of *coconsciousness*, separate, organized centers of attention, receiving impressions and able to be communicated with, in control of the personality (as in the somnambulisms or fugue states) or capturing a leg, arm, or the functions of eating. (The distinction was not between conscious and unconscious or between ego and id, for each hysterical function had its own consciousness, organizing principles, and capacities for communication; the hysterical ego, like the personality, was already split) (Havens, 1973).

Somehow the notion has persisted among some of Sullivan's students that he derided hysterical patients allegedly because they made him feel uncomfortable. (Does any psychiatrist feel comfortable with a "paranoid schizophrenic?") This notion may be due, in part, to the fact that Sullivan's irony often makes psychiatrists uncomfortable themselves. In any event, a close study of his ideas about hysterics does not reveal any lack of respect for this phenomenon. Maurice R. Green has cited two major contributions of Sullivan in regard to the understanding of hysteria. First, Sullivan did *not* separate the dynamisms of the hysteric from the rest of the latter's personality. Second, Sullivan interpreted the dynamisms of the hysteric to an earlier developmental level: the juvenile era. Hence, one must be meticulously accurate in one's exposition of Sullivan's interpretation and treatment of hysterical patients.

Sullivan said that the hysteric might be said, in principle, to be a person who has the "happy thought" as to a way by which he can be respectable, even though not living up to his standards. But the hysteric, Sullivan wrote, does not have such a thought. Yet, this formulation is misleading. Sullivan claimed that the hysteric can often be led *under hypnosis* to recall just the thought that was the key to how one can "dissociate" with comparative impunity and still without anything like the elaborate apparatus of the *true* dissociative condition.

The collision of aspects of the personality involved in the self is said to be also somewhat more obvious in the hysteric than in the more obscure mental conditions (such as schizophrenia). One can observe that the whole achievement or enterprise of the dynamism employed by the hysteric is to prevent the environing people from recognizing and being able to prove the existence of the impulses which are hidden behind the hysterical facade or which in other words are dissociated. Sullivan (1956) said that in the *great dissociative processes* there is *no* awareness at any level of the evaluation that other people might place on the dissociated system. "That is all blotted out in the readjustment within the self-system which gives security by virtue of the dissociation." The self-system of the hysteric is said to be so sketchy that as soon as the other person hits on a fairly well-aimed guess as to what the dissociated impulse is, then the whole business shifts. A new self—against—impulse process is developed and the old one abandoned. Therefore, hysteria is very much simpler than massive dissociation, in which such impulses as the homosexual or hate are buried. There is no "high grade" conflict between ideal structures or moral systems and unregenerated impulses but just a "happy" idea which is "dissociated" of how to get away with something.

Conversely, Sullivan claimed that in the true dissociative processes, as in schizophrenia, there isn't any analogue of anything like that at any time. Hysteria is a disorder of interpersonal relations which results from extensive amnesia.

In *Conceptions of Modern Psychiatry* (Sullivan, 1953), several dramatic maladies, such as the anaesthias, are mentioned, but we will omit them. It is a well-known fact that a hysteric can unwittingly "convert" or "represent" his emotional problems by fits, fractures, paralyzes, and a considerable number of other organic like manifestations. But he is not faking. There is an excellent list of hysterical maladies in Sullivan's *Conceptions of Modern Psychiatry* (1953).

The following illustrates how an idea triggers the hysterical dynamism. A man with a strong hysterical predisposition has married for the sake of money. Owing to his rather dramatic and exaggerated behavior, his wife soon realizes that practical considerations led him to marry her and however distasteful or distressing this insight may be she cannot completely blind herself to her lack of importance as a wife in her husband's life. "So she may begin to get even." She may, for example, develop a "never-failing" vaginismus which makes sexual intercourse virtually impossible. But, a man who has a hysterical predisposition, and the lack of objectivity in interpersonal relations which accompanies it, will not consider that the vaginismus has any relationship to what he says and does. Suffering terribly from the sexual deprivation, he goes to rather extravagant lengths, a certain rather theatrical attention to details of sexual behavior rather than a thoughtful effort to understand his relationship with his wife. But he fails "again and again." And, this lack of success, is not likely to endear him to his spouse. One night, "when he is worn out, and perhaps had a precocious ejaculation in his newest adventure in practical psychotherapy, he has the idea, My God, this thing is driving me crazy" (Sullivan, 1953), and goes to sleep.

Sullivan points out that the idea, "This thing is driving me crazy," is the "happy idea that the hysteric has." But sometime during the night or early morning he wakes up, probably when his wife is "notoriously" most soundly asleep, and has a frightful attack of some kind. Perhaps he has awakened with a cry, clutching his wife in an excess of fear, quivering, stammering. He may leap about, tearing his hair, beating his forehead. This behavior will inevitably awaken his wife, very much frightened. So she calls the doctor. "But before the doctor gets there," Sullivan asserted, "the husband, with a fine sense of dramatic values, will let her know in some indirect way that he's terribly afraid he is losing his mind" (Sullivan, 1956). As for the physician who has been called, he prescribes a sedative and the patient is lulled to sleep. The man's attacks will recur now and then. (Sullivan thought that the continued use of hypnosis increased the probability that the patient will be more disabled and more inextricably hysteric.) "The more dramatic roles," he said, "that a hysteric takes onto himself, the less chance there is of finding the person (behind the roles) and a way of life that is adjustment" (Sullivan, 1956).

Essentially, what the idea "My God this thing is driving me crazy" unwittingly means is "My wife and her vaginismus are having a bad effect on me." Nevertheless, the "happy idea," "My God this thing is driving me crazy," provides him with a way of punishing his wife, although he is not conscious of it. But there is another element to be considered. His lust is "tainted" with his security, although he is not conscious of this either. Since he is strikingly self-centered, everything he does is important, apart from his deprivation.

His verbal formula is directed toward the achievement of a more or less foreseen goal — except that it becomes very swiftly inaccessible to consciousness. This is said to be a much simpler process than a major dissociation, wherein a vast number of perceptions and thought have to be controlled. By "forgetting" the happy thought or event, the hysteric can keep the connection between symptom and "life" obscure. So, the hysterical dynamism works relatively nicely.

Predisposing Factors

The interpersonal behavior of a person with a major dissociation, as long as one takes into account his dissociated behavior, is said to be behavior of a highly sensitive, highly differentiated personality. The person must be capable of remarkable alertness and rather competent, because he has to be warned in time of possible disaster. Otherwise, in integrating situations, his dissociated impulse — which might be hate or a complex array of homosexual tendencies — will result in grave consequences. One can see from what has been previously said that the dynamism of hysteria is, in a sense, much simpler than schizophrenia.

The following characterizations of the hysteric have offended many clinicians. According to Sullivan, the hysteric has a rather deep contempt for other people. Sullivan said,

> I mean by this, that he regards other people as comparatively shadowy figures that move around, I sometimes think, as audience for his own performance. How does this show? Well, hysterics may be said to be the greatest liars to no purpose in the whole range of human personalities. We are not talking about pathological lying (a pathological liar does not believe in the reality of his own experiences). We are talking about the fact that nothing is good enough as it is (Sullivan, 1956).

His conversation undergoes improvement in the telling of whatever it is about, since he has to exaggerate everything a little. His language is said to be twisted in a characteristic fashion. The hysteric describes everything that interests him as he tells it. Apart from their personal life, some hysterics who are highly intelligent can give an objective report of various matters. "But when they talk about their living — their interests and their fun, their sorrows and so on — only superlatives will suffice them." This is Sullivan's ironic way of saying hysterics are rather contemptuous of mere events and mere people because they act as if they were accustomed to something better, "and they are" (Sullivan, 1956).

Development of the Hysteric Disposition

Sullivan held that the early juvenile and late childhood eras in the hysteric are characterized by fantasies of a rather crass dramatic type. This becomes more significant when one realizes that the markedly sensitive, shy, difficult "pre-schizophrenic" might engage in more fantasy than would the person who is outstandingly predisposed to hysteria. The reason is that the schizophrenic has much more time—a lifetime, to devote to fantasy.

> And in the fantasies of the markedly introverted person, who might easily have major dissociations of personality later, one finds that there is a constant growth in the nicety of referential detail; a myth-like daydream of last year would be just too crude to be entertained this year (Sullivan, 1956).

But, "in the case of the person who is developing the hysterical predisposition, a type of fantasy which served his purposes in late childhood may continue to be maintained five or six years afterwards, unchanged except for an elaboration of the characters and possibly a concealment of too glaring and socially unacceptable elements of the drama" (Sullivan, 1956).

One might wonder why the fantasies of the hysteric are so crude and lacking in subtlety in contrast to the markedly introverted person. Sullivan's answer is that the organization of the self—and in Sullivanian psychiatry one must never forget the structure of the person's self dynamism—in the markedly introverted person is a constantly growing, a very urgently and imperatively and necessarily growing instrument for more and more microscopic analysis with a view to more and more foresight of possible rebuffs and pains from other people. Although a markedly introverted person may be painfully shy and appallingly incapable of "handling" other people, he becomes more and more capable of being forewarned so that he may have some possibility of avoiding rebuffs. (In *Personal Psychopathology* Sullivan [1972] provides an exquisitely detailed description of the introverted way of life in contrast to the extroverted, which seems to be more congenial to most Americans.)

The introverted person's purpose is to spot the rebuff in time, if he can, and either protect himself from it, or, failing that, leave. Sullivan claimed that as a result the most private processes within awareness undergo a development to meet this need for ever-increasing scrutiny.

> And the daydream that stirs a little feeling of anxiety—the feeling that perhaps this is not quite the daydream that other people would think was nice—is constantly modified to make proper deferential gestures to certain standards of propriety which, this introverted person has now caught onto, are other people's values. So the fantasy constantly becomes more and more refined and more obscure about primitive things (Sullivan, 1956).

Is it any wonder that Sullivan has been compared to James Joyce? In a very simple sense, Sullivan said, the hysteric is self-absorbed, the sort of person who is often popularly characterized as chronically indulging in "wishful thinking." All sorts of interpersonal "prehensions" or rudimentary perceptions of the self-absorbed are said to be fogged into what is called wishful thinking. The self-absorbed person has no grey. For him everything tends to be black *or* white. A life-long series of potentially educative events has left his capacity for fantastic, self-centered, illusion utterly unaffected. A person whom he dislikes is simply impossible. When he "loves" someone, he is so melodramatic that he confounds the object — unless the latter also suffers the self-absorbed syndrome. His prototype is said to be sought in early childhood (Sullivan, 1953). This description may merge with what Kerenberg describes as pathological narcissism (Kerenberg, 1975).

In contrast to the introverted person, in the person who is predisposed to hysteria and increasingly manifests hysterical symptoms which to a degree are similar to the self-absorbed, there is a disturbance "of the clarity of connection between other people and pleasure or pain." Other people are unimportant to him.

Thus, hysteria is a mental disorder to which the self-absorbed are peculiarly liable. There seeeems to be an overlapping of the two except that the self-absorbed syndrome pertains to a relatively uninterrupted career-line, while the hysteric is more subject to episodic changes in direction of the career line owing to the vicissitudes of his interpersonal relations.

Characteristic Interpersonal Relations

An unsophisticated person may be deceived by the episodic seemingly enthusiastic "happy" and charming behavior of the hysteric. Sullivan (1956) said:

> The observable interpersonal relations of the prevailingly hysterical person are characterized by an extravagance of emotional color. Euphoria is higher than an appraisal of objective reality would seem to justify, and it alternates rather vividly with equally extravagant negative emotions . . . Moods come and go as fleetingly as summer showers and there is no close relationship between the prevailing mood of an hour, let us say, and what might be described as the most important personal events of that hour.

Sullivan went on to say that the hysteric can be very angry, immensely pleased, very devoted, and very hostile in rapid succession. In the hysteric, the maturity of the motivational system is quite incomplete. Since the proportion of hysterics who have not progressed through preadolescence perhaps is considerable, their relationships with people are never ones which amount to love or intimacy (collaboration). The competitive motivation of an hysteric which persists from the juvenile era can be striking, often with members of the same sex — and not rarely with members of the opposite sex. No wonder he (or more likely she) has a "rather bad time" of marriage.

Here is perhaps the most intelligible explanation of Freud's Oedipus Complex. Sullivan thought that the sexual relations of the hysteric are often badly marred by immaturity, and disorders arising from genital impulses, he added, are so common that they account for the libido of orthodox psychoanalysis' being indistinguishable from a generalized lust. The therapist who searches for what is the trouble with the sex life of the hysteric, encounters the crudest expression "of Oedipus survivals." In this connection, one might expect to find the female who hates her mother and is "all but obviously" still very devoted, very firmly attached to her father. One will also discover wives suffering from the hysterical syndrome who make invidious comparisons of father and husband that are derogatory to the latter. An analogous situation obtains in the case of the male.

Owing to limitations of space, Sullivan's amusing but interesting account of treatment of the hysteric will be omitted (Sullivan, 1956).

OBSESSIONALISM

Apart from schizophrenia, the greatest headache an expositor of Sullivan psychology and psychiatry faces is his interpretation of "obsessionalism." In *Conceptions of Modern Psychiatry* Sullivan (1953) stated: "Interpersonal situations including an obsessional person are characterized by obscure power operations directed to the maintenance of control over everything that happens." In *Clinical Studies in Psychiatry* (Sullivan, 1956) the emphasis on power operations has shifted to power over others due to the patients anxiety. Consider two rather obsessional people who are married who consult a therapist. The first one will tell him: "Well the longer we go on together the more crotchety and difficult so-and-so is getting." Sullivan (1956) then added:

> And the crotchety and difficult part proves to be that, as they grow insecure about their relationship, they get to pestering each other more and more in what sometimes seems to be a never-ending effort to, in some obscure fashion, get the other person down. And yet the one does not want to get the other down in order to lift himself by standing on the other's fallen body or anything like that; instead, each one wants to overcome the other's power to produce anxiety — to make the other fellow impotent to produce anxiety.

Since the lectures which have been compiled under the title of *Conceptions of Modern Psychiatry* were delivered in 1939, while *Clinical*

Studies in Psychiatry were delivered in the mid-forties, it seems very possible that the reformulation is due to a much greater understanding of the "obsessional" in the later series of lectures.

In any event, what follows about the obsessional syndrome contains some modifications from the rest of this chapter. For example, we include some illustrations of Sullivan's therapeutic technique which provide a clearer understanding of the obsessional person.

Since everyone who has studied abnormal psychology probably is familiar with the vast array of signs and symptoms which obsessionals manifest, we are not going to try to list them. Signs are said to be phenomena which the clinician can observe more or less directly. But, symptoms must be reported by the patient, since only he experiences them. However, Sullivan developed great skill at building inferential bridges between the two in relation to uncommunicative patients. The distinction between signs and symptoms is vitally important because when the interviewer (therapist) observes a sign he must then inquire whether there are corresponding symptoms which are experienced by the patient. Needless to say, he will need skill in this and other sorts of inquiries. Failure to inquire, which sometimes has to be done in an oblique fashion, may cause the therapist to confuse a genetically determined sign with some psychological (mental) occurrence.

If we use the term "cause" loosely, we can say that for Sullivan, the emotional experience which causes or provokes obsessive thinking and compulsive, ritualistic behavior is anxiety. It is not fear (although anxiety and fear sometimes combine), nor hatred, nor anything else in the human emotional-motivational systems. But, it is also true that anxiety tension can and often does get linked up or associated with a number of different sorts of emotional experiences. But, the fundamental purpose of the psychiatrist is to help the obsessional patient to get rid of the anxieties which often destroy his interpersonal relations and his peace of mind, although this is not the whole story. A reorganization of one's interpersonal relations entails a reorganization of personality structure.

Because some clinicians make no clear distinction between anxiety and fear, some of the differences must be emphasized, as previously pointed out. Anxiety is always related to interpersonal relations, whether the latter be actual, or imaginary, or a blend of both. As a general rule, anxiety is evoked by the actual, anticipated, or imagined disapproval of others, especially significant others: parents, friends, colleagues, lovers, spouses, etc. But it also happens that one may do something or experience something of which one's own self dynamism disapproves, this too may evoke anxiety or what some clinicians might call guilt. This seems to be caused by the fact that one's self has developed in people's transactions whose values and norms for living one will have learned.

Even the most highly individuated person cannot escape this, though he may learn to modify some of those values and norms or to create new ones. It is extremely important to note that anxiety interferes with alertness in one's interpersonal relations so that one fails to perceive or to understand important factors in one's interpersonal situations, including one's own attitudes, feelings, thoughts, desires, and actions.

Fear is said to be aroused by two sets of factors. One set has to do with any threat of injury to the biological integrity of the person. The other set of factors pertains to the actual or anticipated experience of too great novelty. In contrast to anxiety, fear usually increases one's alertness. It also tends to mobilize one's energies—quite in contrast to anxiety.

In *Clinical Studies in Psychiatry*, Sullivan (1956) claimed that both fear and anxiety may be so extreme that they "amount to" terror. He held that it is absolutely necessary for the clinician to determine whether a given patient is suffering from one or the other or a combination of both. Does the terror derive from anxiety because the patient is afraid of something erupting into consciousness? Or, still again, is the terror due to something that is actually threatening and dangerous due to external circumstances. In this case, the clinician must endeavor to bring as much clarity as he can into the "formulation" of what it is that is so fear-provoking. Such a discrimination is vital. If one is to calm a terrified psychiatric patient, for example, the clinician must carefully apply his skill in discriminating what is projection on the part of the anxiety-ridden patient and what could easily appear to be actually threatening. Failure to make the discrimination has the end result of psychiatric and meaningless jargon, as well as destroying what contact existed between patient and therapist.

The behavior of the obsessional person, including the obsessional neurotic person, is designed to maintain a tolerable measure of interpersonal security, that is, to ward off or minimize anxiety. Of course, we are referring to the behavior wherein other persons are involved, not to problems in mechanical systems, engineering, mathematics, etc., where there may not need to be any close personal relations. The "obsessional business" is wholly of the self. According to Sullivan, it has nothing to do with the satisfaction of impulses that do not require the intervention of the self. For example, obsessional phenomena have nothing to do with sexuality *except* in so far as it has been made a source of insecurity; and this "conditioning" of lustful behavior was, at least until recently, apparently quite common. In fact, Sullivan thought that in an obsessional neurotic "the field of lust" is almost always badly complicated by obsessional, ritualistic behavior. But the latter does not produce impotence or frigidity. The obsessional is said to be relatively free or uninhibited in actual genital cooperation, although he may produce "a lot of nuisance" for the other person, regarding his security needs. And it is well to remember that the pursuit of satisfactions and the pursuit of security are often intertwined, interrelated. This can also, in many instances, make things difficult for many who are not obsessional but who also have endured a good deal of unfortunate life experiences.

Sullivan made a distinction between a prevailingly obsessional personality and one who is definitely neurotic. The difference, however, is one of degree only. The prevailingly obsessional person does not impress ordinary intelligent, reasonably observant people whom he comes into contact with as being in all odd or queer. However, with the people he is chronically integrated with, he manifests a definitely obsessional stickiness, a certain type of security operation. The person who gets into this obsessional stickiness with *anybody* who attempts to have any sort of slightly meaningful contact is labeled an obsessional neurotic. The latter is said to be a person who cannot enter into any acutally meaningful relationships without obtruding into an otherwise presumbaly informative, communicative situation, the sort of thing perhaps best described as the "stickiness of obsessional preoccupation."

The stickiness is a form of adhesiveness or tenaciousness in a situation which exerts a sort of compulsion on the other person. As a prototype, Sullivan mentions the stutterer who makes use of language not for communication but for defiance and domination. If one asks him a question, he will set out to answer it. But he does not give a direct straightforward answer. He employs a magic of articulate sounds which really works. By demonstrating an inability to produce a word, and to desist from making it, he immobilizes the other person and "arrests" the flow of activity. Sullivan offers another illustration which may be helpful at this point. Suppose you require a badly needed item of information very quickly which is in the possession of your obsessional secretary. If you urge her to hurry and procure the information from the files, you may convert her into "a mass of jitters which closes off everything." In order to get the information needed, you must wait patiently until she gets through talking about something that is perhaps entirely irrelevant or uncommunicative. There is said to be no way of hurrying things. A frontal attack would be worse than useless.

The therapist has to be conscious of the fact that *miscommunication* is an outstanding trait of the obsessional neurotic. The latter can produce — verbalize — something that sounds very reasonable if one does not try to find out what is really being said and what it may refer to within the framework of obsessional operations. Nor is that all. The obsessional neurotic may employ, over a vast field of interpersonal relations, somewhat meaningless thinking about life in the sense that it is definitely not simply communicative thinking. And Sullivan believed if one cannot formulate an idea in communicable language, one does not understand that idea. Parenthetically, the verbal magical operations of such a person may have their roots in late infancy and early childhood.

It may be asked: What basically ails the obsessional neurotic? Sullivan asserted that the obsessional is warding off and will be eternally warding off, unless he is cured, a type of inadequate self function, which has a long history. Related to this inadequate self function is the fact that the obsessional neurotic has never had the satisfaction or fulfillment of outstanding success in interpersonal relations. The inadequate self function is most clearly manifested in his vulnerability to anxiety.

> His self system has functioned to avoid a great deal of severe anxiety that he knows from experience he could suffer, and, as it were, to maintain a low level of well-being or, to put it another way, a very mild state of anxiety which is a background to some very vivid satisfactions (Sullivan, 1956).

So, he experiences intense anxiety only when the other person with whom he is related is of genuine significance, such as a spouse. He also experiences severe anxiety occasionally because of anticipated satisfactions, but more generally because of past satisfactions with the significant other. This is where the inadequate self-function comes in; or more simply put, low self-esteem allied to an immature self.

Sullivan offers the following illustration. Suppose a person who is quite important to the obsessional neurotic as a source of satisfaction may begin to find fault with the obsessional *not* in the genital field, rather in much less dramatic but more time-consuming areas of the relationship. And this, for the obsessional, becomes a source of anxiety. For the partner begins to wonder why she (or he) has to get "sort of wrapped up in sticky flypaper several hours a day" whenever they engage in sexual relations. The insecurity of the obsessional has generalized, as it were, to areas involving sexual relations. So the obsessionalism gets "thicker," more intense, but he is not able to analyze the situation or do anything about it, because he cannot transcend the limitations of the self and its warping functions. He becomes, or has already become, more anxious and feels compelled to employ magical (incomprehensible, possessing no logical order, having no discernible causal sequence), frustrating performances.

Should it happen that both parties are obsessional, and one seeks help from a psychiatrist, it will be revealed that each one wants to overcome the other's power to produce anxiety. Under therapy, the obsessional neurotic is said to go through motions or behaviors that suggest he is getting absolutely panicky at the prospect of having something clearly formulated in the realm of his personal problem (Sullivan, 1956). According to Sullivan, as the motivational pattern becomes more and more difficult to disguise by security operations, it takes on an aspect of novelty and crosses the line into fear. This is said to be true regardless of what the motivational pattern is—it can even be an estimable one. At that point, the patient tries desperately to bring everything to a halt, that is, "to arrest process." Thus, if the therapist "closes in" on a probable hypothesis, the patient gets greatly disturbed. "As soon as you start anything of that sort," Sullivan (1956) said, "the obsessional practically gets up from the couch and throws it at you—he does almost anything to stop you from talking." He makes it very difficult for the therapist to formulate the problem. And when, despite his efforts, the therapist has stated the problem, the patient gets angry. But he also benefits markedly from the confrontation since, as time goes by, the anger fades away and the interpretation has brought insight or understanding of what was previously so threatening. Of course, the timing of such an interpretation has to be taken into account.

Obsessional states are substitutive processes. The latter are designed to prevent one from ever becoming clearly conscious of something that would be anxiety provoking. Selective inattention seems to be one of the most common of these stratagems. Substitutive processes may run the gamut from deliberately talking about something else, in the sense of changing the subject, to the utmost absorption in intense preoccupation with covert processes, such as fantasies. They are by no means, however, confined to obsessional neurotics. Consider the hypochondriac, whose preoccupation with his illness represents pure substitution for something that would be much more disturbing.

Sullivan has stressed that the more anxious the patient gets, the more he tends to employ magical verbal operations, that is, unintelligible, uncommunicative statements owing to causes already mentioned. Even if they sound communicative, they are not formulated in the syntaxic, consensually validated mode. Hence, whatever reference to "reality" they may have, it is obscure, recondite. In other words, statements by very anxious obsessional people tend to be more or less autistic, or, in other cases, misinformative, miscommunicative, and misleading.

A brief mention of a few outstanding occurrences in the development of the obsessional may be helpful at this point. Very early in his life, a person discovers that verbal statements have rather remarkable power to handle some of the situations that are attended to by anxiety. In some homes, no matter what aggression anyone perpetrates on another, there are always some worthy principles available to the parents, let us say, to which appeal is made. To make matters even more confusing for the child, 15 minutes earlier an appeal to an entirely contradictory principle was employed by the parents. Others may call them hypocrites. But hypocrisy serves a very useful function, because without this limited verbal magic, the only other thing they could manifest would be an "awful lot" of fairly open hostility and dislike and hatred.

Sullivan asserted that in a good many homes of that sort, love was perhaps the only thing that was of no importance in establishing the marriage. Even if one of the partners had not learned this spurious appeal to ethical principles in order to excuse all sorts of selfish, domineering and self-seeking performances, he (or she) will have learned these things by the time the child had come along and learned to walk and talk. So he has a pair of poor parental models. But, even though he learns that a great many patterns of behavior he has picked up do not quite work with anyone, he also learns they are better than nothing. Since he is surrounded from infancy with an almost pervasive verbal magic, he inevitably takes it for granted that this is the way the world is. Of necessity, he has no frame of reference which would help him separate truth from falsehood, consistent relationships from those which in fact are inconsistent to a high degree, factually correct statements from illusory verbal propositions. Thus, he has to learn the verbal magic and the disguised, masked misleading performances, although he has an unclear suspicion that nothing works very well.

Sullivan claimed that to the extent that the verbal magical operations are better than nothing, the patient actually is inhibited from developing some of the most valuable aspects of verbal implicit operations (that is, clear, analytic thinking, foresight, etc.). In particular, during his developmental course from childhood onward, he is prone to bog down in any serious interpersonal problem by his concentrating on this half-satisfying verbal magic which does not really save him from anxiety or greatly enhance his euphoria although it does, or may, arrest severe anxiety and ward off punishment (Sullivan, 1956).

Obsessionalism takes root during late infancy and early childhood, when verbal and other magical operations are ordinarily most pronounced. It grows, expands, and becomes ever more complicated as the youngster proceeds toward chronological adulthood. He will have missed a great deal of experience necessary for successful, contented living. By the time the obsessional is a chronological adult, he will have developed a formidable repertory of obsessive-compulsive operations. His overt behavior will probably manifest a rich complement of rituals, avoidances, etc., which are designed to minimize anxiety.

Sullivan contrasts sublimation and obsessional operations. He defined sublimation as the unwitting substitution for a behavior pattern which encounters anxiety or collides with the self-system of a socially more acceptable activity pattern which satisfies part of the motivational system that caused trouble. In more fortunate circumstances, symbolic processes occurring in sleep are said to take care of the rest of the personality (Sullivan, 1953). In contrast, obsessional operations are clumsy, uncomfortable, mildly or even severely disturbing performances, which leave one less secure than he was previous to the anxiety-provoking occurrence. The very business of turning one's energy into the obsessional dynamism consists in giving oneself a very mild jolt, a reminder that 'that doesn't work because,' so that one does not feel quite as secure as one did before the disturbing situation arose. Summarily, the obsessional neurotic is not an "unutterably jittery" person, intensely anxious, with profound inferiority feelings. He is not a prey of paranoid grandeur. His self system functions to avoid a great deal of severe anxiety and to maintain a low level of well being.

Having presented a skeleton outline of Sullivan's theoretical formulations of obsessionalism, in order to round out the picture, one must try to present a summary, however limited, of his ideas on therapy. He had no sympathy, he said, with ultra-refined interpretations of the particular verbal content of the obsessional's productions or the particular pattern of a ritualistic gesture. To be sure that verbal content means something to the patient, something that is likely to be more or less autistic, and therefore one cannot perceive the meaning very clearly, if at all. "But what of it?" Sullivan said. The verbal behavior of the obsessional is not employed to communicate; it is employed to obstruct and to protect oneself from suffering anxiety or more anxiety. Trying to seek the original, historical meaning is probably useless, since there is no necessary evolution from an originally meaningful context. (In various lectures, Sullivan asserted that this historical reconstruction is the only way one can understand a particular pattern of bizarre behavior with some patients.)

Tic-like movements and automatisms are said to represent action necessary to maintain a dissociated system when there is no indication for organic etiology. But even though it may be very hard to get an automatism to unfold into what it represents, it does stand for something very important. But, Sullivan did not think a direct attack on its origins is necessarily the easiest way to discover what the therapist is seeking. He taught that he sometimes found, in treating "obsessional schizoid" people who had automatisms, that as certain of the patient's problems were cleared up, the origin of the automatism would become clear to the patient. The latter would report

> wonderful and sometimes immature types of thinking which were to him an adequate explanation of the automatism, even though they were not very meaningful to another person. In other words, such things as automatisms are built by types of implicit activity that are pretty young (derived from childhood experience), so far as our ordinary acquaintance with them is concerned (Sullivan, 1956).

This suggests Sullivan's discovery that some patients whom he had treated shift back and forth between obsessional and schizophrenic symptomatology. It follows that a psychiatrist who is treating an obsessional must be careful not to put too much pressure in the area where the patient can't stand it. It is now thought that many patients who present with a severe obsessional symptomatology mask schizophrenia.

The following is a basic assumption of Sullivan's ideas on therapy with the obsessional. One does not strike *directly* at the self-esteem of an obsessional neurotic. Nor can one hurry his insight very much, although he is pursuing it in his own way. The patient wants to get well. In fact, the clinician must know that until his interpretation of a particular life situation has become almost self-evident to the patient—and this follows usually after a lot of hard work—there is no use in trying to offer any interpretation. Otherwise, the therapist may spend a month going around in circles. For the obsessional neurotic, this can lead him on a merry digression. If the clinician does not get in the patient's way—by premature or precocious interpretation, for example—and if he does not prod the patient in some way sensitive region, what occurs is that the context under discussion is being repeatedly run "through the mill," through the patient's mind. And each re-run, makes things a little clearer than they were the time before. According to Sullivan, that is how obsessional personalities seem to heal themselves.

> They run through their security operations over and over and over—but not entirely without the rest of the personality achieving something in the process, for each time the context gets a little clearer (Sullivan, 1956).

Obsessional neurotics are not knowingly malicious although they may seem to be. Furthermore, they have no great difficulty in seeing through statements almost always made to them by people involved with them to the effect that they are terribly difficult to live with, that they are "awful companions." Therefore, they are apt to take time out in self-pity and these "excursions" in therapy and in everyday life are intensely obsessional. The obsessional neurotic who *cries*, cries from rage, and his self-pitying performances are said to be invariably thoroughly designed to crucify someone else. Sullivan asserted that there is a lot of what can easily be interpreted as hostility because this is an attempt to maintain an uncertain security which has to occur all the time when anyone who is significant is around. So, the obsessional who has to maintain a feeling of security while experiencing a marginal feeling that the other person does not respect him is not apt to be loving. As far as *the other person* is concerned, the obsessional seems to be hostile or malevolent.

The recitations of the obsessional neurotic about the past are said to come gradually to reflect brutality toward the patient by a significant other person, usually a parent. Sullivan thought that if this recital of brutality includes some thin disguise which the parent wore, the therapist may always accept the account as being reasonably close to the truth, namely, the very cruel parent always wore a mask to conceal his (or her) brutality. The obsessional learned that his parents were not happy with each other and that at least one of them was savagely cruel to him while wearing a constant thin veneer of convention and sweetness. The latter baffled the child so much that he took to wondering whether the parent was really cruel or whether the parent was filled with sweetness which his own perversity made to seem cruel. We surmise that this may be a possible origin for the ambivalence found in later life in the obsessional patient.

The relevant part of treatment is said to consist in the patient's coming to see—gain insight into the fact—that all the conventional sweetness was just a veneer. Thus, in the process of injury, what was mask and what was motive becomes somewhat clear. Bitter grieving (which may be healthy or sometimes morbid) may attend this insight. In general, the patient grieves over the countless number of opportunities he lost. The lost opportunities, which may have occurred over a long period of time, at first originated in the patient's bafflement as to whether he was right or wrong about the savage interference of his parent. Sullivan adds that this insight, attended by normal grieving, constitutes the final emancipation from a lost object which has been festering, as it were, in the personality since childhood (Sullivan, 1956). Sometimes morbid grieving occurs which may result in a severe depression. This entity is also described today by the term "pathological grief reaction."

Sullivan has some ideas on psychosomatic illness, more specifically disturbances of the viscera frequently associated with obsessional personalities. These too we must pass over. They are discussed in *Clinical Studies in Psychiatry* (Sullivan, 1956) and in *Conceptions of Modern Psychiatry* (Sullivan, 1953).

Obsessionals are said to have a genius for getting all sorts of things involved in their situations, although only for the purpose of befogging troublesome and inescapable situations. Even so, a good many of their satisfactions are sought with "almost blatantly simple directness." The simple directness is quite often beyond their control, since that is all the devlopment they ever had to make in a particular area. But, Sullivan claimed, obsessionals are not as well socialized with regard to certain of their needs for satisfaction as some people. The pursuit of satisfaction and of security are intertwined. So, if someone points out what crude creatures they are in a particular situation—designated as "dating"— they are helpless. Like a squid, they extrude a cloud of confusing details where everything becomes nebulous at the threat to their feebly supported prestige. And, if their therapist attempts to work on these confusing details, he is wasting his time and his patient's time and money. Sullivan taught

> that if one could really keep one's eye on the ball with these people, they
> would not neccessarily be such remarkably slow therapeutic prospects. But
> it takes a high degree of alertness to sort out quickly what is relevent and
> what is merely convenient fog (Sullivan, 1956).

Otherwise, the therapist becomes entangled in all sorts of irrelevant and immaterial objective techniques. He becomes furious at the patient's foggy arguments. And the latter reciprocates. And, within 15 minutes, neither therapist nor patient knows what is going on. The therapist may think that his patient is shifting the topic, misunderstanding everything he says, ascribing the most astounding meanings and lowest motives, etc. to him. Thus, the psychiatrist, who does not want to waste a lot of time, will not quarrel with an obsessional neurotic. If he does, he will encounter another of the patient's befogging procedures. But the latter, in this instance, instead of employing all sorts of irrelevant extraneous details about his life situation, is picking up all the irrelevant and immaterial internal or subjective details that he can find or suspect in his therapist, who is now an antagonist. And the patient's attributions in some obscure fashion have some vague relevance to the personality of the therapist. Sullivan says that explains why they keep on so that the therapist becomes quite entangled. Hence, both are furious and frustrated.

It will provide some perspective on obsessional states and operations, to recall that the obsessional neurotics almost never live in a really tender, considerate, and constructive environment. One might almost claim that their life experiences have precluded it, as well as their own current shortcomings. Hence, healthy, contented people probably veer off from them. The obsessional is said to show a marked tendency to get involved in a situation which can be very crudely described as hateful. Although Sullivan would not offer such an appraisal to his patient, he often used it for orienting his own investigation. He would seek to discover how the significant and helpful other person—the patient's spouse, for example—failed, how his efforts at communication or intimacy miscarried. Sullivan would start out blandly with the observation that certain things are not working out too well—as revealed perhaps in an initial interview or series of interviews—and one might be able to discover what the other person does which gets in the way, even though it is well or very well intended. As a result, the patient usually revealed entanglements, a situation in which things go from bad to worse (Sullivan, 1956).

In these entanglements, husband and wife, for example, engage in mutual *miscommunication* and mutual recrimination, so that resentment between the two increases rapidly to the point of considerable hostility and frustration. Such exchanges leave both parties quite disturbed and baffled.

In the interview, Sullivan would explore such an exchange by asking his patient what happened, who said what next, and then what followed that up. The patient, as he reports, and recounts, may think that his therapist is trying to discover just what kind of a polite she-devil her husband is living with. But what the therapist is trying to do is to obtain data that are "somewhere near" what actually happened. He may often hear what the other person actually said, and a great deal of what the patient said. But, the latter will unwittingly omit some quite important data. A number of things which the patient contributed, that show how the "melée" started will not be mentioned. This indicates how the "melée" became more and more inextricably unprofitable. And it is almost a certainty that many illusory me-you patterns (parataxic distortions) had entered into the exchange between the patient and his spouse, "lover," or whomever. For such causes, early in the interview series, the therapist will almost never get an accurate picture of what went on. But, when he does obtain some notion of what went on, he may depict it in rough outline for the patient to hear—provided the latter has some general outline himself and is not bogged down in parataxic distortions. Otherwise, Sullivan reported what he had heard, except that he did not depict his suppositions of the patient's contribution to the melée. But, the latter will perceive that the picture of the picture of the melée reported back to him is not right, even though it is an accurate reflection of what he said. So, he becomes disturbed at what he thinks must be an unfavorable impression the therapist must have of the other person. Sullivan would then ask just what is wrong with his impression, which he does not think is such an unfavorable one; he is simply reporting what he heard. Since the patient is not satisfied, he attempts "to fix the story up."

As he reformulates the story, Sullivan would do nothing except to ask questions about something he did not understand. The new formulation of his story by the patient may provide clues as to his part in the flypaper operation. And if a clue shows up, the therapist is apt to mention it. This is one of the places where Sullivan's therapeutic enemy—the self-system—comes in. If the patient is quite frequently and noticeably anxious, the therapist will choose comments with very great care, because he is trying to circumvent the security operations of the patient's self. Thus, if the opposition is very strong, he would *not* give any sign early in the therapeutic relationship that he doubts the completeness of the story he heard. He has to "go easy" in warning the patient that he is trying to catch on to what occurs in his entanglements. Sullivan adhered to the general principle that a therapist must not say or do anything which will make his patient more anxious—except for very good exceptional cause. Sullivan first adopted this principle when treating schizophrenics and subsequently did not greatly modify it, although he recognized that, at times, one must say or do things which stir up anxiety or the patient might ramble on forever. Be that as it may, when the patient does not pay much attention to what the therapist may think, it is suggested that he had so much confidence in his obsessional substitution that he would not be unusually disturbed in communicating with the therapist. So, then the latter may ask questions which are close to requesting what he really wants to know. In *The Psychiatric Interview* (Sullivan, 1954) these techniques are explained and expounded at length.

In the course of time, namely, as the interviews proceed, the patient will report something from one of these entanglements that is succinct enough and unguarded enough for the therapist to be able to say "Oh and then you said so-and-so? That was kind, wasn't it" (Sullivan, 1956). Since what the patient had said was quite *unkind,* Sullivan's irony would start some verbal fireworks. Then, he sat tight until calm was restored and the patient began to wonder what was so unkind about it. So Sullivan repeated his statement in the face of his patient's attempt to attenuate the impact of his unkind statement to his spouse or whomever. "Now," Sullivan would add, "I don't see how that could do other than hurt the feelings of your wife, do you?" And in almost all instances, the patient would reply, "No, I don't. I think it was unkind." In this fashion, perhaps over a series of interviews, the patient discovers that, "far from being utterly long-suffering and hopelessly misunderstood and just not up to the standards of the other person, he has taken extremely shrewd blows at the self-esteem of the other person (Sullivan, 1956).

After a few clarifying exchanges of this sort between the patient and his therapist had been "accumulated," Sullivan thought he was somewhat near to doing therapy. The problem of finding out how these melées start could be tackled. Next time the patient reports a difficulty with his protagonist, Sullvian was apt to begin, "Oh, well, just let's get this entirely straight from the start. Just exactly when did you get home, and how had things been going at the office?" The therapist wants the patient to portray a little of the background for the difficult occasion first. Then he wants to know when the background events and the diffiuclty were "met." And after that, the point is brought up when something happened to trigger the difficulty. At this step, obsessionals always want to recite a multitude of detail unless the therapist intervenes. In brief, Sullivan would abruptly say, "Well, what did you make of that remark of your wife." But almost invariably the patient cannot make anything out of it. So he responds with a question. "What do you mean?" To which Sullivan would say, "Well, come now, can you recall when this remark was made to you?" Usually he cannot. Then Sullivan would persist as follows:

> Well this is how something began. Now I gather a lot followed it, but this is really the start of it, and I think that that remark would have called out some feeling. Three or four different things have occureed to me as possible meanings of it. What occurred to you? What did you think your wife meant by this remark? (Sullivan, 1956).

In this fashion of "hounding" the patient, Sullivan could usually extract a statement—a recognition—to the effect that his wife's remark was hard on her husband's self-esteem. Afer saying that that was one of the ideas he had too, the therapist would ask: "Tell me what on earth do you suppose brought that out?" Once more the patient wants to recite a plethora of details—and is cut off. "No, no, I want to get clear at the start and then I'll be happy to hear the details. Now you have been all through all this, and you may have some clues." Does the patient have any clues as to what his wife was getting at by "taking a crack" at him when he arrived home from the office? Again the patient "resists" by an attempt to report what followed the wife's insulting or offensive remark. Now that Sullivan has "closed in" on the patient's resistances, the latter reveals that his wife's remark was quite unfriendly, something which made him anxious, disturbing his self-esteem. And the therapist would "polish" this revelation, making sure there could be no doubts about the wife's unfriendly statement which triggered another one of the husband-wife quarrels. After that the therapist wants to hear the rest. "Ah yes, well it sounds very reasonable to me. Now go on, if you will, with what you can recall of the account." But, the rest of the story is greatly condensed. This is because once the original wound, the spouse's attack on her husband's self-esteem, is laid bare, the patient no longer sees much sense in repeating, or reenacting, the vast waste of time which has been consumed in showing no hurt feelings but nevertheless retaliating, even if indirectly, by various stratagems—all of which occurred entirely unwittingly.

In preparation for the next step, Sullivan "documented" that on a few occasions the patient was not very kind to his troublesome companion, and, similarly, that the latter on a few occasions had started trouble with "very shrewd punctures" in the vulnerable, tender areas of the patient. Then, the therapist is in a position to comment on the "amazing amount of resentment" that must have "piled up" and festered in *him* from having absorbed his companion's rather inconsiderate, anxiety-provoking performances. After listening to a running, complicated opinion from the patient, Sullivan makes the next move. He comments on how much resentment must have piled up in the spouse, only as a result of his shrewd, if somewhat delayed, perhaps indirect, blows at her vulnerable, tender areas which aroused anxiety, resentment, etc. The patient may find this harder to take, but he usually does. And then the therapist can "wonder" out loud: "Why is there so much obscure dissatisfaction in the relationship?" This is followed by other questions before the patient has a chance to deluge the therapist with more grievances, rationalizations, etc. "How is your wife really of very definitely constructive value to you?" This is what Sullivan is really looking for: the constructive values in the relationship between husband and wife. Often, despite reportedly daily warfare, real assets appear in the account of the companion or spouse by the patient. And it is not difficult to infer from this that the patient has assets which are appreciated by the companion or spouse. Although there is a justifiable basis for the relationship, a good deal of warping, humiliating, and attacking exchanges between the partners has been chronic.

Now, Sullivan is in a position to inquire into the original source of the destructive parataxic distortions combined with frequent quarrels in order to undermine a way of life which has existed for years. "What on earth can be behind this? It looks to me as if both of you must be carrying on in the long phase things that belong somewhere in the past, not with each other. Let us see where in the world these patterns begin..." (Sullivan, 1956). This very long "build up" was required if the therapist may expect a reasonably rapid, revealing of the role of the significant parent, usually the mother, who, as Sullivan used to say, "provides the basic patterns of being human." In "our type of society," the significant parent is the mother, because father spends the greater part of his working life away from home earning a living for his family. Nevertheless, in varying degrees, as we know, the father can and does contribute toward a benevolent or malign influence. This is followed by juvenile society, etc.

In this ironic fashion, Sullivan asserted that, by dint of discovering how the patient suffered from the mother's kindly and constructive efforts on his behalf, he could finally say, as if by accident: "God, was there anything that you did of which your mother unqualifiedly approved?" At first, the patient struggles to get rid of this totally unexpected suggestion. But, within a few weeks he will agree that he cannot recall any, unqualified unexpected approval from his mother (and/or his father). So what could his attitude toward his mother really have been? How could he have avoided hating her?

By this time, Sullivan is probably well into the Detailed Inquiry outlined in *The Psychiatric Interview*. When necessary, he will resort to relatively free association. Over the long haul, a great deal has to be worked through. If feasible, the patient's obsessive-compulsive way of life will be markedly attenuated whether or not it can ever be completely eradicated. But, if all goes well in the long run, he will emerge from therapy with a vastly improved repertory of interpersonal relations and perhaps a considerably developed ability for intimate exchange with a fellow human being.

REFERENCES

American Psychiatric Association, Task Force on Nomenclature and Statistics. DSM III — Diagnostic and Statistical Manual of Mental Disorders 3rd. ed., Washington, D.C., APA, 1980.

Havens, L.L. *Approaches to the Mind*. Little, Brown and Co., Boston, 1973.

Kerenberg, O. *The Borderline Condition and Pathological Narcissism*. Jason Aronson, New York, 1975.

Nemiah, J.C. Conversion Reaction, in Freeman, A.M., Kaplan, H.L., and Sadock, B.S. *Comprehensive Textbook of Psychiatry III*. Williams and Wilkins, Baltimore, 1980.

Nemiah, J.C. Psychoneurotic Disorders, in Nicholi, A.M. ed., *The Harvard Guide to Modern Psychiatry*. Harvard University Press, Cambridge, 1975.

Randall, J.H., Jr. *Nature and Historical Experience*. Columbia University Press, New York, 1958.

Sullivan, H.S. *Conceptions of Modern Psychiatry*. 2nd ed., W.W. Norton, New York, 1953.

Sullivan, H.S. *The Interpersonal Theory of Psychiatry*. W.W. Norton, New York, 1953.

Sullivan, H.S. *The Psychiatric Interview*. W.W. Norton, New York, 1954.

Sullivan, H.S. *Clinical Studies in Psychiatry*. W.W. Norton, New York, 1956.

Sullivan, H.S. *Personal Psychopathology*. W.W. Norton, New York, 1972.

7

Schizophrenia and Paranoia

In certain of his lectures, Sullivan said that the schizophrenic experience is approximately equivalent to the nightmare. But, in schizophrenia, the person undergoes this nightmarish experience during waking hours (Sullivan, 1956; compare Bowers, 1974).

According to Sullivan, the essence of the schizophrenic state is a failure of the self-system to reserve attention for the types of referential process (thought processes) that enjoy good repute among the intelligent. Or, as he also said, in the schizophrenic state there is a failure to restrict the contents of consciousness to the higher referential processes that can be consensually validated.

It may be well to recall that there are many gradations in the level of refinement of referential processes. "At one end of the scale are the referential operations of very early life in which there is no precise delineation of what is really relevant and important in achieving a satisfaction which is itself unknown or very dimly realized: such a state of mind might be described as a vague and global feeling of unutterable turmoil (Sullivan, 1956). In any event, the infant's experiences first occur in the prototaxic mode. As he develops, it seems doubtful if there is any day or week in which discriminations begin to be made in his experience. Sullivan conceived of the parataxic mode as a state in which rudimentary discriminations predominate, but are neithter logically nor factually connected. Thus, over a period of approximately 15 years, a person of normal or superior intelligence progresses from a state in which the most rudimentary discriminations are lacking, through many gradations at which the level of thought processes is increasingly refined by an ever more exact realization of what is actually relevant to the result that one seeks. However, the higher one goes on the scale of refined referential processes, the less of life is relevant to him. For example, a physicist or a mathematician employs very rigorous and elegant thought processes when he publishes a new theory. But, this may happen once or twice in a lifetime. Of course, intensely gifted—and sometimes competitive—

physicists spend much of their working lives in a laboratory where high level thought processes are also required. (See Bleuler, 1913, 1950, and Arieti, 1974.) At the very pinnacle of refined referential processes are those "ideational operations", which pertain to mathematico-logical thought processes, a cognitive processes which, in a fashion analogous to Plato's Essential Forms, are independent of the everyday world of physical and social life (Arieti, 1974).

Paradoxically, under certain circumstances such as waking reverie, dreams, and nightmares, one may drop back (regress) at it were to an earlier level of intellectual development. Very early in his career, Sullivan delivered an unpublished lecture and still later in *Personal Psychopathology*, in both of which he asserted that people generally do vastly more "fantasy thinking" than rigorously logical and consenually validated thinking. That is one reason that an average politician can almost always defeat a professor should he run for the same office. The former understands thoroughly the thought processes and emotions of his audiences which the latter may, although understanding the citizen's best interests, blunder innocently into making erudite speeches. As Sullivan said, it is pointless to interrogate a Republican or a Democrat as to the real (and perhaps temporally remote) causes of his political allegiance. James Reston, the brilliant editor and columnist of the New York Times, pointed out a few years ago in a column on the opened page, that the Democrats had been running pretty successfully for about 30 years against Herbert Hoover.

The schizophrenic process is said to take a place with the referential operations of very early life. "There is not the most rudimentary discrimination between what is relevant and what is irrelevant in a vast total situation that is impinging upon one's end organs (Sullivan, 1956)." This is the prototaxic mode of experience. Sullivan added that, correspondingly, there is an extreme lack of clarity as to the action which reaches the goal (any goal), if it is reached at all. As previously implied, cause-and-effect thinking as to why the goal is or is not reached is utterly lacking.

SCHIZOPHRENIA, PARANOID STATES, AND RELATED CONDITIONS

Conceptually paranoia and schizophrenic disorganization may be conceived as being at two opposite poles. Yet, Sullivan claims that everyone who gets lost "in the schizophrenic morasses" has paranoid feelings and may be led to express paranoid content at times. Conversely, every "paranoid" that Sullivan encountered has a period of some schizophrenic disorganization in his history. As we know, the person who presents a paranoic picture blames others for feelings of his own which he cannot tolerate. In order to make this plausible to himself, he develops very highly systematized delusions of persecution and grandeur. Sullivan asserted that out of perhaps 3,000 veteran cases with which he had some contact in a hospital (St. Elizabeth's, Washington, D.C.) where he worked for a brief period, he did not discover one patient who approached pure paranoia.

It is not possible to make a "blanket transfer of blame" without the person's reverting to some use of the earlier types of referential processes. Although parataxic referential processes may be tolerated in late infancy and early childhood, subsequently one must learn more refined verbal thinking or "high grade" referential processes which entail verbal thinking. One must learn that not all cows are black, for example. At the same time, as the childhood era progresses, the learning of language, however imperfectly, coincides and coalesces with the basic structure of the self. The earlier, more or less parataxic, thought processes have to be "stamped out" because of the childhood socialization and what is sometimes called "negative reinforcement or punishment."

> Now the doctrine of pure paranoia would require that the person was wholly secure in his psychosis; there would literally from the standpoint of theory, be no necessity for the self, except as a device for keeping track of all the attacks upon one and so on. But so massive a maneuver as practically eliminating the necessity for the self would require something other than operations with the validated verbal symbols which are so intimately related to the self; in other words, the self must be subjected to processes which are not classically of it, and these processes are the early, nonvalidated types of thinking which appear in later life as schizophrenic processes (Sullivan, 1956).

And so Sullivan concluded that it is safe to say that every paranoid person has at some time been schizophrenic for at least a little while. Although this thought may not have been absolutely correct, since the boundaries of the group of disorders labeled "paranoid disorders" and their differentiation from other disorders, particularly severe paranoid personality disorder and paranoid schizophrena, are unclear (American Psychiatric Association, 1980).

The Paranoid Dynamism

The paranoid dynamism has not been sufficiently clarified. Its source lies in (1) an awareness of some kind of inferiority, which then (2) necessitates a transfer of blame on to others. There is another thing which differentiates the paranoid from the schizophrenic. The latter lacks the necessary knowledge and sophistication about people which would enable him to put the blame on others for his own malfeasances. The schizophrenic is very vulnerable to *being blamed* for the malfeasances which other have inflicted on *him*. But, these descriptions constitute only a "paranoid slant on life." (For example, one who is as chronically suspicious of people and inclined to blame them for one's own mistakes and shortcomings.)

But, a third factor, must also occur to reach a "full-blown paranoid state," namely such a misinterpretation of events that it amounts to an explanation "usually transcendental" in the nature of whatever is troublesome. The people around one are viewed as devilish. But, the person does not move to California or even Florida if he lives in the Bronx or Brooklyn. He remains where he is, even though the people among whom he lives may have "created an exquisitely built-up plot to injure or destroy him." The following abbreviated account of a patient Sullivan interviewed better illustrates the "transcendental" nature of a "paranoid's" delusions.

> On entering the office, and seeing me make it safe from eavesdropping, he drew me an an odd diagram on a piece of paper. This, he explained, was the symbol of an association he enjoyed with a scientist with whom he had had a casual contract on one occasion, abroad. I learned that these two people were about the most important people on earth. They exercised vast powers achieved by command over natural forces, through the instrumentality of hypnotism, and were soon to achieve what we now know as the ambition of Mr. Hitler, hegemony of the world. They were in constant communion, across the continent, by telepathy. Both were imperiled by a horde of secret agents who were all around us. In brief, the patient revealed a well-systematized paranoid state, with but incidental schizophrenic remnants in its structure. He revealed it because, he said, he had received an unmistakable command to do so immediately (Sullivan, 1953).

The manner by which one reverts to primitive thought processes is not very recondite. Sullivan asserted that one reaches back to late childhood when significant people blame us at times, taking out on us their disgruntlements with their own carelessness, their lack of judgement and various other things, including, perhaps, some harsh treatment or painful rebuff by an envious neighbor. The parents were unfair, and if one dared to attack their unfairness, they "compounded the felony" by denying it. rationalizing, etc. Although their defense of the unfairness amounted to a double offense, it also provided one with a measure of reassurance "for we know then they were very inferior people." If the parent, or some other person, cannot admit a fault, he is obviously not as secure as he seems. Thus, everyone has experienced something like this: "I wouldn't have this horrible feeling of discomfort with others if *they* weren't there, and if I hadn't been educated the way I've been educated by other people

(Sullivan, 1956)." One can also think the following, which at times was true in ones earlier years: "And I wouldn't have this sense of discomfort if other people didn't treat me unfairly."

But blaming others is not "bomb proof." Someone who is skeptical of one's penchant for blaming others may demand solid evidence for his idea that he is being wretchedly treated and unfairly blamed for all sorts of things. And, as Sullivan might say, this can be very awkward.

To achieve the paranoid dynamism, one must achieve another thing which was previously outlined. This is the "rather transcendental explanation" of why people blame and persecute others. However, the greater the feeling of insecurity one has, the more risk there is of schizophrenic processes appearing. In that case, the refined cognitive processes of the self system begin to weaken and so one's level of mental processes is in danger of sinking disastrously, to a more primitive level and disorganize.

Paranoia and Homosexuality

Freud had the notion which he arrived at by a technique more suitable to the literary arts than to science, that paranoia is due to repressed homosexuality. It happened that a German magistrate, Daniel Paul Schreber, after having spent 10 years in a mental hospital, was discharged and in 1903 published a long narrative of his delusions. On the basis of this narrative, Freud published a "pathography" of Schreber. Ellenberger (1970), in a cogent summary tells us:

> Among all these delusions (of Schreber), Freud singled out two particular ones that he held as fundamental: First, Schreber contended that he was in the process of being changed from man to woman; second, he complained of having suffered homosexual assaults on the part of his first physician, the neurologist Flechsig. Freud assumed that repressed homosexuality was the cause of Schreber's paranoid illness. Schreber's homosexual love object had been his father, then Flechsig, later God or the sun . . . Fundamental in the delusions of persecution was the mechanism of projection. The denied sentence, "I love him" was replaced by, "I do not love him." "I hate him . . . because he hated and persecutes me."

Sullivan thought that Freud's association of paranoia and homosexuality is not only misleading, but dangerous to therapy based on this association. The paranoid process is, to a high degree, the result of incomplete development of personality during the preadolescent and adolescent eras. In order to illustrate this idea, Sullivan summarizes the "case" of a boy, a preadolescent, whom he worked with intensively. "This boy," he said, "had an appalling life." The following is an illustration: Apart from someone very early in life, who treated him like a human being for a brief period and who "finally escaped" from the boy's home and, despite her pity for him, left the boy to suffer, everything else that happened to the boy is said to have been as unfriendly, frustrating, and savagely cruel as one might expect from the then prevalent theory of schizophrenia. In school, he was a holy terror. During chronological preadolescence, he made the disheartening discovery that "all the available kids" toward whom he might have been friendly fought shy of him, apparently because they were impressed with "his problem character." The pathos of his experience during this time is revealed by the fact that he attempted "by serious application and much disciplinary planning" to convince his potential chums that he was "human" like themselves—but he failed. Had there been another "sick" boy more or less like himself present in the school society the two might have teamed up, but there was not. "And lo, he came out with a fine paranoid system" (Sullivan, 1956). For example, he would entertain the other unsuspecting boys with a fictitious story of how he was really a very important person who had been stolen as an infant from the hospital for reasons of blackmail by the person who claimed to be his mother. Moreover, this boy had fabricated an elaborate amount of pseudo-data to provide proof of his story.

According to classical Freudian theory, the youngster "bogged down when he thought of moving toward women, owing to his intense hatred of his mother." This lady had been extremely cruel and thwarting toward him. Since the mother may be considered—perhaps with reservations—as a "symbol" of womanhood, he had an intense barrier toward women—so the classical interpretation might run. As adolescence approached, one might theorize, the boy suffered an intense homosexual conflict. Sullivan (1956) asserted,

> But in my simple minded world it is a little difficult to talk about homosexual conflict where there is no homosexual attachment. What he had was an inescapable barrier to intimacy with man, woman, or beast—as a matter of fact, he had no pets; part of the thwarting business was that the mother would not put up with his having any animals in the house. (Sullivan, 1956).

The once famous formula: "frustration breeds aggression" is too simple to apply to this "case." In any event, the boy managed to live as best he could, given his incredible (but not so rare) experiences in the home, becoming an extremely difficult juvenile, hated and feared by teachers, "and quite a gifted thorn in the home situation." When he matured to the point of requiring intimacy with a fellow human being, he failed abysmally. Repeated failure at his efforts to achieve intimacy ultimately forced him to conclude, "They would have no use for me." This thought was a conscious conclusion of a recurrent theme, "I am too inferior to get what I must have." Such a reflection is so intolerable that the boy finally reached the solution of blaming others, with the necessary supporting secret evidence of why he was persecuted. Perhaps, needless to say, this "solution" cannot work at a conscious level.

In general, according to Sullivan, when the psychiatrist studies any "paranoid" who is moderately accessible or about whom one can get highly relevant historic data, one discovers no reason to suppose that the patient had progressed *through a patterning of* sexual behavior before the appearance of the paranoid state. On the contrary, the investigator (psychiatrist) discovers that such a person was defeated in establishing workable sexual habits. It is this final defeat which constitutes the situation in which the paranoid development appears.

Sometimes, Sullivan added, the clinician discovers that these people have had a pretty satisfactory preadolescent experience in the sense that, although they were warped, they still in some distance progressed toward securing intimacy. That sort of experience may have been possible to them, in case they were badly disturbed, because there were other quite disturbed fellows with whom they could establish a relationship, which, however imperfect, was much better than none. In other instances, the psychiatrist may find that "paranoids" may have had a good deal of the benefits of an intimate relationship with an older person who did not really pay much attention to what was going on. Still, again, if such unfortunate people were not badly warped, they may have been fortunate enough to be intimate with a person for a time. Sullivan said, "But then, they bumped into the business of comporting themselves like other young men, which too often in this culture means abandoning real happiness in favor of heterosexual prestige" (Sullivan, 1956). Summarily, it is the need for intimacy conjoined with the inescapable awareness of a fatal incapacity for that intimacy that evokes "this desolating paranoid dynamism."

The Remainder of the Personality and Sleep in Paranoia

The person who suffers this desolating paranoid dynamism cannot maintain a conviction of self-esteem in connection with significant others. It follows that there must be serious deficits in the satisifications which require the cooperation of others. Therefore, there has to be an extraordinary effort to use "symbolic tools" during sleep in order to diminish the tensions of unsatisfied needs. Otherwise, there would be a collapse of the self.

Sullivan asserted that before the appearance of the paranoid development, the sleep function will be rather badly disturbed and there will also be waking evidence of a good deal of dissatisfaction, tenseness, and perhaps motivation which does not seem to get itself applied any too well. Somehow or other, the person initiates something but he does not persist in pursuing it. His diminished self-esteem complicates the feeling, so that he believes he could not get whatever he wanted from the other person. Sullivan (1956) said,

> For example, let us say that a heterosexual situation starts out showing many traits that are identifiable as an attempt on the part of the man to effect a sexual relationship with the woman. But, the situation moves rather unpleasantly into a twilight zone where the drive toward sexual gratification is no longer so clearly the purpose of the thing; and out of this certain twilight it becomes a matter of his quarreling with the woman as to whether women are really any particular good or whether they are entitled to take themselves as seriously as they do about sexual choice, and so on.

As one reflects on such a situation, it is difficult to know whether the man was seeking a fight or sexual intercourse, because the ultimate test is the "end state." This man started out apparently for one thing and wound up with another. This sort of unhappy occurrence may happen in many kinds of situations, due to the failure of the self function. "In consequence, the unsatisfied person has all sorts of dream processes and one thing and another, remembered or otherwise; and then comes the paranoid development" (Sullivan, 1956).

The sleep of the paranoid, while it can be seriously disturbed, is said to be by no means as bad as it was before the paranoid state appeared. Although he may report that his sleep is just as badly disturbed as it ever was, the objective observer will find that the paranoid's sleep is distinctly better. But, every now and then, it is said to be definitely interrupted by dramatic dream experiences which are more or less consonant with the general persecutory trend. Although the psychotic content manifests itself as dream processes, these dream processes are of a piece with waking dream processes. Therefore, he identifies them as actually valid. Sullivan claimed that dream processes of such a patient are not different from the latter's waking experiences, such as many of his exquisitely complicated misinterpretations are, which constitute his orientation in living.

The improvement of the sleep function that is said to come with the paranoid development tells the psychiatrist a good deal, including something more of the dynamism of hate (Sullivan, 1956). Sullivan explains this as a kind of pseudo-sublimation—a pseudo-sublimation in the sense that in the paranoid development the person wants to integrate a particular type of satisfactory situation with another person except that this type of situation has always made him intolerably insecure as to the other person's esteem for him. Thus, the only way he can attain any satisfaction of his desires it to combine them with the pursuit of security by a hostile, derogatory method. And, this method is not calculated to include the reigning Hollywood beauty—whoever she may be—to walk hand in hand with any man.

With regard to the pseudo-sublimation, which is the "solution" of many impulses previously frustrated, and which provides partial satisfaction, Sullivan's speculation is elaborated more fully as follows. He surmised that the original paranoid thought was,

> I want to be close to this person for a feeling of warmth which I need because I'm lonely: but if I move toward him he will regard me as inferior and unworthy and will deny me this warmth because he won't warm so inferior a person. By a slight shift in the original pattern it becomes: That person wants to be warmed by him so that he can injure me by refusing. He is a hateful enemy (Sullivan, 1956).

A malevolent transformation seems to occur. Nevertheless, a remarkable amount of time is said to be spent in all but closeness to this person, sometimes in acutal physical closeness to him, and sometimes, Sullivan asserted, the warmth is sought in a rather subtle way, so that it may be given. Paradoxically, the consciousness of the paranoid person is that of hateful derogation of himself by the very person who provides warmth.

Sullivan summed up the paranoid person's interpersonal relations by his assertion that such a person obtains partial satisfaction of integrating tendencies (needs, motives) by making the attitude of the other person hateful, projecting a hateful motivational system onto anyone with whom he is related. Still, very few can stand the punishment he radiates for long.

> In other words, paranoids are persecuted by everybody from whom they want warmth, and therefore the particular person who happens to be involved in the paranoid situation at the moment is only a respresentative of society, which is very easy to generalize (Sullivan, 1956).

THERAPY OF SCHIZOPHRENIA

Once more, because of the vital importance of schizophrenia, we depart from the usual order of exposition. It is important to remember that in Sullivan's view, the clinician should determine whether homosexuality is the organization of a definite integrating tendency or drive that satisfies a need, or whether there is a complex mental disorder in which the homosexuality is present because it so perfectly "fortifies some abnormal mental process, some dynamism of difficulty." Sullivan asserted

> where a person has felt that life is eminently worth living only in the preadolescent stage, when he did enjoy intimacy with another person of the same sex, irrespective of whether that great intimacy was what may be described as on the non-genital or the genital level, I am quite willing to deal with that person on the basis that he is engaged in actual direct pursuit of satisfaction from members of his own sex, or in homosexuality, as it may easily be called (Sullivan, 1956).

But, if such experience is missing from a person's life then, according to Sullivan, one is doing a great violence to the therapeutic principle should he accept the notion that the person has anything like a simple drive to secure genital satisfaction by any type of behavior with a member of the same sex. Sullivan thought that to work on this assumption, and to attempt to deal with such a patient's "homosexuality" is, he asserted, one of the most vicious miscarriages of therapeutic situations. The therapist destroys any possibility that he can establish any intimacy or rapport with the patient. In effect, the psychiatrist is saying, "abandon all hope of feeling of personal security and then we might be able to do something." Since the patient has previously acquired the belief that there is a revolting difference between him and good, respectable people, the clinician is reinforcing the patient's conviction.

Hence, it is very necessary to differentiate between (1) the isophilic or preadolescent phase of personality development and the satisfactions that can be acquired during that era; and (2) the countless unhappy caricatures of living to which clinicians sometimes apply the term homosexuality. Sullivan claimed that the people who have gotten well into the preadolescent phase of personality development before possibilities of further growth failed, and who come to psychiatrists with their life problems formulated in terms of homosexual concepts, are still somewhat closer to reality. Conversely, the people who seek help from psychiatrists and who have not progressed as far as the preadolescent phase of personality development while formulating their problems in terms of homosexuality, are manifesting a much more complex distortion of interpersonal relations and offer a much more treacherous basis for therapeutic relations, because they are much less mature. Here is a vital key to prognosis in therapy: How far has the patient progressed in the course of his development?

THE CATATONIC: THE ESSENTIAL SCHIZOPHRENIC PICTURE — IN CONTRAST TO THE PARANOID AND THE HEBEPHRENIC

Sullivan asserted (Note: For Harry Stack Sullivan the true schizophrenic state is the catatonic.) that persons who suffer a schizophrenic disorder and who are apt to wind up as chronic paranoid patients, are statistically apt to date their onset from much later in chronologic age than are the durable catatonic states or the hebephrenic. According to Sullivan, the essential schizophrenic state is the catatonic. Traditional categories are largely due to the errors of Kraepelin, who was a great categorizer. However, it may be Sullivan was not quite fair to Kraepelin (Havens, 1973). Sullivan emphatically stated: "The distinctions between paranoid schizophrenia, paranoid states, and paranoia will not, I am sure, stand up under any very intensive study of individual patients" (Sullivan, 1956).

The currently published Diagnostic and Statistical Manual of Mental Disorders (DSM III) (American Psychiatric Association, 1980) leaves this question still unanswered. Schizophrenic disorders are classified separately from paranoid disorders. The limits of the concept of schizophrenia in this manual are stated to be still unclear, but the approach taken utilizes clinical criteria that include both minimal degree of chronicity and a characteristic symptom picture. The boundaries of the group labeled paranoid disorders and their differentiation from other disorders, particularly severe paranoid personality disorder and schizophrenia, are stated to be still unclear. The classification used in DSM III includes in the class of paranoid disorders — paranoia, shared paranoid disorder and paranoid state (American Psychiatric Association, 1980).

With sure strokes, Sullivan paints a developmental outline of catatonia and hebephrenia.

> Let us assume that one encounters very grave conflicts between one's needs for satisfactions and one's necessity for feeling secure and free from severe anxiety long before there has been a consolidation of intimacy with a fellow being, a real other person. Then, if there is a schizophrenic disaster — that is, loss of the control of awareness (consciousness), with the eruption into the field of attention of less refined and specific referential processes which might be called dream thoughts or reverie processes ordinarily ignored — this will be followed by a course which quickly eliminates from the manifestations of the self a great many of the recent additions of the self (Sullivan, 1956).

The gross picture of the hebephrenic includes a strikingly regressive course — deterioration — in which speech habits, social habits, and social values usually manifested in behavior, dilapidate to an indefinitely specifiable level or to a state that is similar to a wholesale organic deterioration. Sullivan thought that there was no way of discovering whether the intelligence factors swiftly deteriorate as well.

For the sake of comparison and contrast, let us compare the person who has experienced intimacy with a chum during the preadolescent era. Then, should he become schizophrenic, it will not bring about so swift a deterioration. Sullivan thought the schizophrenic disaster will follow a course primarily characterized by its close relationship to the nightmares which are experienced by adolescents and by some chronological adults.

> In other words, the conflict between the need for satisfaction and the need for security lowers the threshold of awareness to the point where these processes escape the excluding device of the self system and take the place of the finely focused referential processes (Sullivan, 1956).

This conflict is said to have a great deal to do with the very thing one sees in troubled dreams and nightmares, which represent the highly sustained application to the solution of a problem "of rather high orders of reverie processes and subverbal or autistic verbal operations."

But, if any time the patient despairs while undergoing the nightmarish experiences of the catatonic state the hebephrenic change (dilapidation) may occur. But there is another possibility instead. The catatonic patient, if he despairs, may arrive at the paranoid solution so that he evolves into paranoid schizophrenia or the paranoid state.

The Catatonic State

The patient, as a self-conscious person, in the catatonic state, is profoundly preoccupied with regaining a feeling of security of the kind rarely manifested after early childhood. Or more exactly, the "integrations" which the catatonic seeks are like those in which a person under three years of age might be involved. What may be still more confusing to the psychiatrist, is that an indefinitely great part of the relevant experience which the patient has undergone over a period of years continues to be evident. The integrations mentioned above include parataxic illusions after the pattern of the Good Mother, the Bad Mother, the Good Father, the Bad Father. To the extent that acculturation subsequent to childhood is still effective, it provides the illusory people (Good Mother, Bad Mother, etc.) with various attributes said to be derived from religious beliefs and/or the particular mythology which the patient has learned.

The following tells what kind of experience catatonics underwent a generation ago. The experience which the patient undergoes is of the most awesome, universal character: he seems to be living in the midst of struggle between personified cosmic forces of good and evil, surrounded by animistically enlivened natural objects which are engaged in ominous performances that it is terribly necessary — and impossible — to understand. He is buffeted about. He must make efforts. He is incapable of thought. The compelling directions that are given him are contradictory and incomprehensible. He clings to life by a thread. He finally thinks that he is dead: that this is the state after death: that he awaits resurrection or the salvation of his soul (Sullivan, 1953). Ancient myths of redemption and rebirth seem to reappear, not, according to Sullivan, because the patient has tapped some racial unconscious, but owing to the fact that he has regressed to a state in which only an early type of abstract thinking can survive. "He is dead but clearly not through with life. . ."

While the catatonic patient is undergoing these dreadful experiences, he shows no interest in the commonplace acts of living. He does not eat or drink. He pays no heed to excretory processes; nor does he talk and appears mute.

He does not recognize the personal meaning of other people's actions in his behalf. He may show little activity: may lie nude with eyes closed, mouth finally shut, hands clenched, most of the skeletal muscles in a state of tonic contraction. He may engage in strange, often rhythmical, movements. He may undergo sudden eruptions of excitement, occasionally pass from must catatonic stupor into violent excitement with seemingly quite random activity. . . (Coleman, 1972).

The Evolution of the "Paranoid Schizophrenic State"

Sullivan went on to consider a case in which a personal orientation of the awesome phenomena is found. Suddenly, the patient "understands" it all: the spread of meaning, magic, transcendental forces, etc. as the doings of some other concrete person or persons. This is said to mean that the schizophrenic state is taking on a paranoid coloring. If there is a marked diminution of the suffering of the patient as a result, one observes the evolution of a *paranoid schizophrenic state*.

Sullivan thought that this evolution is of a much less favorable outcome, since it tends to characterize *permanent* distortions of interpersonal relations; although the unpleasantness of the patient's experience gradually fades and a quite comfortable way of life may ultimately follow. Sullivan pointed out that the transfer of blame for the results of one's inadequacies does not remove or reduce the manifestations of the tendencies concerned. But, he said, the transfer of blame decreases the feeling of insecurity and, to that extent, it reduces the probability that powerful tendency systems will escape from dissociation and precipitate conflict, regressive change, and perhaps frank schizophrenic phenomena. Therefore, the achievement of a paranoid systematization is so markedly great an accomplishment in the course of a schizophrenic disorder that it is seldom relinquished.

Sullivan (1953) characterized systematization thus: "One systematizes a belief by suppressing all negative or doubt-provoking instances, and by bolstering an inherently inadequate account of one's experience with rationalizations in the service of an unrecognized purpose." The relatively great improvement in security is, however, accomplished at a terrible price because, after a period of years, most of the patients who have suffered paranoid schizophrenic decompensation, become indistinguishable from the condition of those in whom the hebephrenic change appeared early—perhaps during the incipient schizophrenic state when the patient may appear more and more preoccupied; inattentive; or given to puzzlement, misunderstanding and misinterpretation, as he becomes more autistic and seclusive.

It would be a great mistake to think that the more purely paranoid state is a comfortable way of life, however eccentric the paranoid person may seem to unsuspecting neighbors. Sullivan claimed that the paranoid person must be integrated in paranoid interpersonal relations, that otherwise the power of the dissociated tendencies comes to exceed (as in catatonic schizophrenia) the power of the self to dissociate them with anxiety, conflict within consciousness or panic, and probable eruption of schizophrenic processes. The paranoid person may write bitter and troublesome letters to his Congressman, or start law-suits, or pester psychiatrists, or intimidate neighbors. Since he cannot merely "repose in his persecutions and grandeur," he must do such things.

Paranoid states can become self-fulfilling prophesies. If one examines carefully the paranoid delusion, one can usually find some reality core in it. If the paranoid patient does not have someone persecuting him in reality, after awhile he secures someone to persecute him because of his paranoid behavior.

A typical clinical vignette demonstrating this tendency may be illustrated by the following: A 35 year old paranoid patient was brought to the North Central Bronx Hospital Emergency room in New York City by his family because of extremely agitated behavior. The patient claimed that the president of the United States and the F.B.I. were persecuting him. During the evaluation, it turned out that this paranoid delusion appeared a few years ago during an acute decompensation of the patient's self and since then, the patient has been engaged in writing letters to different authorities including threatening letters to the president, so that the F.B.I. actually began an investigation.

The Hebephrenic State

It is important to point out that, according to Sullivan, there are no types of schizophrenia, only certain fairly typical courses of events in some people's lives who have suffered destructive experiences at the hands of their parents or parent surrogates and others, at least as early as the early childhood era. According to the classical scheme of classification, there were four main types of schizophrenia: simple, catatonic, paranoid, and hebephrenic. These classifications were based on a medical model. Whether the clinician can legitimately employ medical models in the description and explanation of mental disorders is still moot. At any rate, Sullivan thought that a "type" of functional mental illness is not analogous to a physical disease entity. Schizophrenia (catatonia) may suddenly erupt following upon panic (a collapse of the self or disorganization of the personality), which may be due to say, a homosexual encounter, which is violently at odds with one of the person's conscious norms and ideals. Or, schizophrenia may appear gradually, insidiously, which Sullivan thought to be more dangerous, of ill omen, since it implies that the person has suffered grave misfortunes in his personality development earlier than the person who suffers the sudden onset of a schizophrenic episode. The latter has progressed further in his growth. Hence, he is likely to have more assets and abilities, and fewer liabilities. However, the variables in the etiology of any mental disorders are multiple and one cannot be too sure about how much weight any one merits.

It is clear today that there are multiple variables contributing to the emergence of schizophrenic states, although genetic factors have been proven to be involved in the development of the illness, the relatively low concordance rate even in monozygotic twins indicates the importance of nongenetic factors (American Psychiatric Association, 1980). The issue of the relative weight of biochemical versus psychosocial, or interpersonal factors, in the development of schizophrenia is still unsettled (Van Praag, 1976).

Before outlining certain factors omitted in the account of catatonic schizophrenia, we will briefly cover the last — and almost irreversible — state called hebephrenia, wherein the person has apparently divested himself of the human qualities he acquired from very early in life.

The *hebephrenic dilapidation* is the other unfortunate outcome, in addition to paranoia of schizophrenic states. Sullivan said this change may appear very early in the course of schizophrenia or it may occur as the termination of a prolonged catatonic state. In any long-continued schizophrenic condition that has not tended markedly toward recovery it will eventually appear. After a period of years, most of the patients who have suffered paranoid schizophrenic conditions are alleged to become indistinguishable from the condition of those in whom the hebephrenic change appeared early. Sullivan believed that when it appears, the hebephrenic state is apt to prove permanent, although he credits Kempf with the cure of one such patient and the "spontaneous" recovery of a few patients Sullivan had studied.

The outstanding characteristic of the hebephrenic state is a marked seclusion. The hebephrenic avoids any companionship. There is a disintegration of language habits to the point where his speech is described as incoherent, vague, unconnected, or manifesting poverty of ideas. The hebephrenic evidences a marked reduction of emotional rapport. Thus, he gives the impression of dilapidation or impoverishment of the emotional aspects of life. Of course, these characteristics make no sense except in an interpersonal context. Such a patient performs strange, impulsive, and "senseless" actions. In any significant interpersonal context, the manifest mannerisms, hebephrenic or otherwise, come about by the stereotyping of a gesture or some other interpersonally significant pattern of behavior. Such an activity is said to become relatively rigid in the way it occurs, no longer delicately adaptable to the circumstances of the particular occasion. (Various kinds of mannerisms are illustrated in Sullivan, 1953). Sullivan added that to these descriptive features, that these patients suffer vivid but changeable auditory and visual hallucinations and that they entertain changeable, fantastic, bizarre, or "silly" delusions. Beyond this point speculation can be treacherous.

Sullivan's comments on hebephrenic mannerisms include that they appear to be most illuminating. Their meaning is the most remarkable thing about them. "Not only do they represent the autonomous activity of impulses dissociated from awareness (consciousness), but they represent the activity of impulses that were once a part of the self dynamism, the dissociating system. In the hebephrenic state, what remains of the self system maintains more or less of a feeling of security by excluding from awareness various impulses which were a part of the prepsychotic self (Sullivan, 1953). The impulses of the prepsychotic self had a part in the conflict and chaos of the catatonic state because they were in conflict with dissociated impulses previously "unconscious" and more or less subject to control by selective inattention and other strategems of the self. The impulses of the prepsychotic self were still "on the side of the angels" during the catatonic state because they were opposed to the impulses whose manifestations horrified the patient. "Now, they themselves are in much the same relationship to the patient's awareness. If they tend strongly to integrate an interpersonal situation (say, affectionate tendencies), the patient becomes acutely anxious, and often becomes seriously disturbed, perhaps acutely hallucinated, excited, assaultive, and more or less randomly destructive (Sullivan, 1953).

The hebephrenic way of life does not seem to involve the field of human relations — even though some of them may carry on pseudo-conversations with other patients. As a rule, the patient is said to show more effort in avoiding personal attention from others than in anything else. His is not the more familiar withdrawal from discouragement, humiliation, and feelings of being disliked. Because his peace of mind is seriously disturbed by even the most rudimentary relation with any real person, he avoids all semblance of intimacy with anyone. Sullivan claimed that the hebephrenic's regression may be so great that he is aware of very little except elaborations of sentience connected with the physiological processes of his body. Furthermore, all that remains from the long process of acculturation (education in the broad sense) and all that remains of his motivational tendencies, which once provided high gratification is, so to speak, dissociation. The characteristics of a civilized being, in so far as they once existed, if they existed at all, are now expressed mannerisms, that is, "the stereotyping of a gesture or some other interpersonally significant pattern of movement." He has abandoned the troublesome demands of living among people and their ways of life.

It would be a mistake to think that hebephrenia is a state of contented vegetation associated with primitive reveries and the simplest of zonal (oral, anal, genital) satisfactions. It is true that many such patients, if left alone, seem to be content for long periods. But all of them, according to Sullivan, endure long episodes of extreme violence and agitation. The provoking circumstance of such behavior was entirely obscure. At least part of the time, they are busily hallucinated, although the voices were usually endured "in good part" but under some circumstances that were unpleasant and thoroughly disturbing. Moreover, many hebephrenic patients talk with the hallucinated voices,

> have long felt compelled to maintain amicable relations with the illusory "they" whom they hear, and have in fact sunk into the hebephrenic state in gradual relinquishment of any independent existence (Sullivan, 1953).

Sullivan did not know whether once the hebephrenic change has begun, the patient will continue to sink in the scale of personal values, or will finally arrive at a relatively stable condition. This he thought was beyond early prediction. He also thought that if the deterioration continues, the final state of the patient is practically indistinguishable from that of the deterioration called *dementia praecox*, simple type. The latter patients manifest, among other things, a seeming evaporation of any interest in events impinging on them as Sullivan (1953) asserted.

Although catatonic schizophrenics suffer grave demoralization, their situation is not hopeless—provided they receive intensive treatment. One very significant factor, as previously noted, relates to the question of whether the patient had any genuinely meaningful relationship during the preadolescent era. For example, Sullivan said that if a schizophrenic episode occurs, it will be characterized by a much prompter appearance of the hebephrenic develoment than generally occurs in the case of a person who enjoyed intimate preadolescent experience. Preadolescent experience creates a meaningful tie to the real interpersonal world.

> It is the lack of a tie with what one may call the real interpersonal world which is so conspicuously lacking in the hebephrenic, whereas that very tie is so conspicuously troublesome in catatonics and in those who eventually make paranoid elaborations (Sullivan, 1956).

Summarily, according to Sullivan, the onset of catatonia may eventuate, owing to the person's career in (1) a paranoid "solution," (2) hebeprhenia, (3) recovery.

Finally, we refer to the latest integration of clinical and research data regarding the phenomenology of schizophrenia as it appears in the Diagnostic and Statistical Manual (American Psychiatric Association, 1980). "The phenomeno-subtypes are subcategorized in order to reflect the major cross sectional clinical syndromes, despite the knowledge that some are less stable over time than others and their prognostic and treatment implications are variable" (American Psychiatric Association, 1980). This approach is consistent with Sullivan's approach, who clearly stated that he expected changes in the field as our knowledge progresses. Thirty two years after his death, the phenomenology of schizophrenia has not changed drastically. The DSM III allows for "phenomenological subtypes," changes from one entity to the other, only if there is a predominant clinical shift in the clinical picture that persists more than several weeks. In addition, in the DSM III, the term "Disorganized" is preferred to Hebephrenia, although the latter is put in parentheses, the category "undifferentiated" is used when the episode of illness is characterized by prominent psychotic symptoms that cannot be classified in any other category, or that meet the criteria for more than one category at the given time. The authors of DSM III tried to allow for the prognosis-outcome factor by introducing a "residual" category (American Psychiatric Association, 1980). (For an interesting discussion of the topic see Carpenter, 1977). One should note that this approach deviates from the original Sullivanian thinking.

THE SCHIZOPHRENIA DYNAMISM: A REVIEW

The tripartite view raises three questions. What happens to the self? The rest of the personality? And sleep?

The Self

The essence of schizophrenia is said to be a failure of the self system to contain attention to the higher referential processes that can be consensually validated. The inclusion in awareness of primitive, diffuse processes dealing with esentially rather terrifying states of nature occurs. Sullivan asserted:

> In such a situation, for example, I, as a person known to me, would no longer be fixed and relatively durable (as in normal self-continuity) but, instead, would become much more like a toy boat in a real monsoon: and other people would not be the more or less truncated caricatures that I have moved uncertainly among, but would become embodiments of rather terrifying generality (Berger, 1966).

It is the culture mandates, the norms, the prescriptions and proscriptions that one has not been able to live with, which are the things that have become terrifying and generalized in these primitive processes.

What we discover in the self-system of a person undergoing schizophrenic change is said to be, in its simplest form, an extremely fear-marked puzzlement which consists of the use of rather generalized and anything but exquisitely refined referential processes, in an attempt to cope with what is essentially a failure at being human. In other words, the schizophrenic fails in his efforts at being anything that could be respected as worth being.

The Rest of the Personality

The problem of what occurs in the remainder of the personality, once there has been a collapse of the self, is extremely difficult to discover. All ordinary channels of communication are said to be closed or at least are so disordered that they are almost effectively closed.

> You never know whether you have something that is meaningful in the sense that it was meaningful the month before with the patient, or whether you have something that has an autistic meaning, an exact parallel of which would not be found in your own case after you had reached the age of five (Sullivan, 1956).

It has to be taken for granted that the language processes of the schizophrenic are obscure. Hence, getting a valid clue from the patient about anything that is occurring outside the self system is very difficult. Perhaps, one should add that despite such great difficulty, Sullivan became extraordinarily skillful at catching on to what the patient might be trying to communicate.

THE FAILURE OF DISSOCIATION IN SCHIZOPHRENIA

The schizophrenic change is apparently due, generally, to the person's inability to maintain dissociation. This inability may occur insidiously over a period of time or quite abruptly. An example of an abrupt onset will be given from a "case" which of necessity is probably disguised in its superficial aspects in order to protect the identity of the patient.

Sullivan interviewed a young man who had been suffering from a severe obsession state. There was one symptom which bothered him, he said, although he had received sporadic treatment for years previously by another therapist. This young man related that except for one symptom which still bothered him, he was completely cured: He still had to throw away the part of his food which his fingers touched. In the face of great reluctance, Sullivan insisted there must be something which involved another person. Under great pressure, the patient revealed that as a boy aged 10, he had worked in a bowling alley where he first had developed a fear of being poisoned as a result of touching varnished wood. "He had then begun an excessive washing of the hands and an avoidance of that part of a slice of bread and the like which he had handled." Only then, did he reveal that he worked with another boy in the bowling alley. Still under the therapist's insistence, he remembered that he had grown to be great friends with this boy. He recalled that the two had grown to be remarkably intimate; they had gotten to lie in each other's arms and to fondle each other. The patient recalled that he never did it again. He agreed with Sullivan that the worry about touching the wood of the alleys appeared after he had been made to realize that there was something wrong with the intimacy with the other boy—in fact, after he had stopped it.

Sullivan said that since the patient's regular therapist (who had been ill) was not to see him for another six weeks, he did not continue the interviews. However, Sullivan did say that he did not ask the "interviewee," as he subsequently often called his patients, as to the role of his hands in the happy intimacy with his friend, nor as to any physical basis for the idea of poisoning by way of the mouth.

Then again, perhaps because of the necessity of distinguishing a patient's identity, Sullivan said:

> Taking our young man who is assumed to have sublimated all recognized manifestations of lustful, genital, integrative tendencies, let us confront him suddenly with an extremely attractive and most forthright person who firmly believes that lust should be satisfied and that its satisfaction is unqualifiedly good—also, that he is attractive and suitable for genital integration (Sullivan, 1956).

The outcome was more or less similar to that of the episode described below.

Before proceeding further, it is important to emphasize that in a footnote Sullivan acknowledges the unlikelihood of such a consummation. He pointed out in a sort of shorthand, omitting the context of the encounter, that a person who found the young man attractive and suitable for genital integration could not be so healthy.

The young man "succumbs" and enters effectively, although perhaps not wholeheartedly, into the integration. At the moment he has a "shockingly good time." However, it is assumed that evil early experience has done its work, and that, as a result, the aftermath is self recrimination and severe conflict, which may quickly appear. In such matters, there is no exact formula. Something of the young man's state of mind will be communicated to his female partner whether there is any discussion about it or not. An "extemely attractive and most forthright person," who firmly believes that lust should be satisfied and that its satisfaction is unqualifiedly good, would almost certainly know all the symptoms and behavior patterns of the sexually satisfied, normal male. If something seemed awry, she would be likely to ask something like the following: "Is there something wrong, darling? Aren't you happy. . .?"

Let us assume that this man leaves his partner with some hurried words of appreciation, although she may still have the impression that he is in a curious state of mind. By an effort at preoccupation with something else, he will put the thought of his experience out of his conscious mind. But, he sleeps badly the next night, perhaps tossing through the night, bedeviled by unpleasant dreams. He will feel very restless the next afternoon, take a long walk though he feels increasing fatigue. Although he may set out for anyplace, in the course of his walk, and without warning, he realizes that he is returning to see his sexual partner — "that he is burning to repeat the experience." Upon this realization, he is literally terrified. Panic or a state bordering on panic is said to supervene.

Sullivan formulated panic as an acute failure of the dissociative power of the self. His description is superbly graphic. Suppose, he said, that you had walked each day for years across a little bridge in the sidewalk, and one morning it suddenly gave away and sank a few inches under your feet. Phenomenologically, the eruption into consciousness that accompanies this experience — "a blend of extremely unpleasant visceral sensations with a boundless and practically contentless (object-less) terror" is panic.

> All organized activity is lost. All thought is paralyzed. Panic is in fact disorganization of the personality. It arises from the utterly unforeseen failure of something completely trusted and vital for one's safety. Some essential aspect of the universe which one had long taken for granted, suddenly collapses; the disorganization that follows is probably the most appalling state that man can undergo (Sullivan, 1953).

The failure of the dissociative power of the self, which results in panic is in this instance (of the young man whose encounter with the young woman who was an enthusiastic advocate of sexual "sports"), not merely the collapse of a sublimatory reformulation of genital drives due to the evil effects of early life experience. Sullivan asserted that there was also a barrier to women and the corresponding homosexual motivation which existed in dissociation.

He emphasized the shattering nature of the disorganization, which he called panic. Were this state to continue, life would not last long. Apparently, inherently reparative factors still exist after such a disaster as panic. Thus, Sullivan said the personality reintegrates as swiftly as possible; often as a state of terror with extreme concentration of attention on escape from the poorly emphasized danger mentioned earlier in this chapter. "Unless something of this sort is possible, panic eventuates in circus movements, random activity, and finally incoordination of the skeletal muscles" (Sullivan, 1953). The extremity of this state is suggested by Sullivan's statement that the terror-stricken person is all alone among deadly menaces, more or less blindly fighting for his survival against dreadful odds.

Restriction of Perception

There is said to be an extreme restriction of perception which is illustrated by the belief that one is being watched and followed. Many terror-stricken patients believe themselves to be followed by other people at times in automobiles. The explanation seems simple. A normal driver keeps an eye, with the help of his driving mirror, on the cars immediately behind him, as well as watching out for the cars immediately in front of him. In the case of the schizophrenic, all the cars he notices are behind him.

As a car passes, it ceases to have any relevance whatever. It is no longer perceived. Therefore, no car passes one, and so long as there are cars behind one, and they stay behind one, it must be that they are menacing (Sullivan, 1953).

Delusions and Hallucinations

Normally, the auditory zone is closely related to the oral zone, particularly in the "coordinate function" of communication. One has a need to hear and a need to talk, which are said to be manifestations of the tendency to enjoy any ability that one possesses and by the biologically inhering needed to reduce tension by the expenditure of the supply of excitation. Were one deprived of such abilities, the disaster might seem not much less severe than the loss of vision. In the normal person, the major zones of interaction are under the control of the self. In the phase of terror following panic, one or more zones of interaction become functionally autonomous — that is, they are no longer under the control of the self system. It is usually the auditory zone which becomes intermittently autonomous in the phase of terror. Thus, the phenomena of auditory or other hallucinosis

represents the noticed activity of one of the zones of interaction as the expression of a dissociated system. One hears voices, spoken statements which pertain to the experiential structure of the dissociated integrating tendency (Sullivan, 1953).

Such an automatism is expressive of dissociated impulses to integrate some particular interpersonal situation.

Schizophrenia is said to literally mean a fragmentation of the mind, and data suggests that in acute schizophrenia there is a clear fragmentation of perception with response to part, rather than whole percepts (Bemporad, 1967; Avieti, 1964). There is a splitting of the control of awareness. This is in contrast to all other functional mental disorders. In non-schizophrenic states, awareness of the personal meaning of the situations in which one exists is restricted to relationships brought about by tendencies in the self. One is conscious of nothing else except conflict and anxiety. But, in schizophrenic states, awareness includes not only that which is in the self and also "that which attends the autonomous functional activity of the hallucinating zones of interaction." But, all meaningful experiences are referable to the self. Some "buried" system of integrating tendencies included so much energy that they could no longer be dissociated — hence the intolerable conflict. Sullivan claimed

> In schizophrenic states, on the other hand, a state of conflict has as it were been universalized, the conflict-provoking tendency systems being accorded independent personality with power greater than that of the self. Instead of anxiety, there is fear and often terror (Sullivan, 1953).

In so far as the self functions, the patient is said to be engaged in infantile magic operations in an attempt to protect himself, to regain some measure of security in the face of mighty threats, portents, and performances in a world that has become wholly irrational and incomprehensible.

At this point, we will mention something that was ignored in an earlier part of this chapter. The schizophrenic person cannot cease to suffer the terrifying dissociated experiences by accepting them, or assimilating them, as part of the self. To do so would entail undergoing an extensive change in personality, with all that it implies: a marked change in the sorts of interpersonal relations one would sustain in daily living. Nor could one have any foresight as to the direction and extent of the change. There is no way of knowing whether such radical change would be tolerable. Therefore, the schizophrenic person cannot easily reintegrate a unitary awareness, which is more or less tantamount to a restoration of a unified self.

Sullivan also pointed out that the patient cannot accept the manifestations disowned as the performances of others (wherein one or more zones of interaction become functionally autonomous, as in delusions and hallucinations). The patient cannot accept these manifestations, even though "they" communicate abuses and disturbing suggestions to him, who make him have disagreeable and disgusting sensations, who otherwise destroy his peace of mind, and by fatigue and other interferences reduce him to deeply regressed states of being. "Everything in his "personal awareness"—for he now has two—repudiates any suggestion that the experiences are not real, or that they arise from his unrecognized needs and desires (Sullivan, 1953).

Sullivan, on the basis of a great deal of work with schizophrenic persons, held that if a person who suffers from schizophrenia has fortunate experience with the "more real people" (actual people) whom he encounters in his disturbed state, the fury of the hallucinosis may decrease, the welter of delusional perceptions may diminish, and something approximating a stable maladjustment of a deeply regressive sort may supervene. In these fairly quiescent states, the regression of personality processes is said to be such that the patient lives in a world and participates in interpersonal relations, all of which are dream-like in varying degrees.

Sullivan showed that the variations of details in the pattern of catatonic interpersonal relations is great. But, the ideas on schizophrenia outlined in this chapter will serve as a useful introduction for those who wish to pursue this disorder in greater detail.

RELATIONS OF THE SELF-SYSTEM
TO THE TOTAL PERSONALITY

Try to envision a person, Sullivan said, who does many things which are pretty meaningful, but then destroys your belief that you could be right as to what these things mean, by the extraordinary character of the context in which they are carried out. A simpler way to state this is that after doing something that seems pretty meaningful to an observer, the person then does other things which seem to deny completely the correctness of the conclusion the observer has arrived at a few moments earlier. Although such a hypothetical person may not appear to be schizophrenic at first glance, *he does appear very much like what the schizophrenic notices about himself*. Sullivan asserted that the schizophrenic has "this puzzling awareness" that he is doing something he ought to recognize, that sometimes he does recognize it with an excessive terror; and at other times he is just hounded by the fact that it ought to be clear, but that some way or other it eludes him. Thus, in schizophrenia, the self-system is rather nearer in identity to the rest of personality than in any other marked mental disorders. This is due to the fact that the self has no monopoly of awareness, as was pointed out previously.

The sleep of schizophrenics is profound. The "machinery" of the self, its various security operations, including its dissociative funciton are no longer operative. The self-system no longer possesses the instrumentalities to foster the needs for satisfaction in more normal people, including the need for sleep. The schizophrenic does not lie awake fearful, anxious, or excited about a planned journey. But, the sleep of schizophrenics is said to be different also from the sleep of normal people—it is a regressive phenomenon. Such persons may sleep 10, 12, 14, or 16 hours a day (Sullivan, 1953). It is analogous to the withdrawal from reality of "markedly schizoid people" who may sleep 10, 12, 14, or 16 hours, punctuated by brief periods of wakefulness.

Despite expectation based upon associations between dreaming and psychosis, current research shows that the laboratory sleep of a hospitalized schizophrenic is relatively normal. During acute episodes, sleep is often disturbed and dream time is low. It is possible, that this is an effect of extreme anxiety. Some chronic schizophrenics will show perfectly normal sleep patterns, in others slow wave sleep (stage 3 and 4) decreases (Hartman, 1975). Questions remain unanswered in reference to the sleep of schizophrenics, such as the specificity of the rebound failure of schizophrenic after REM deprivation reported in the literature, and the possibility of sleep disturbance factor operating independently of psychiatric diagnosis (Zarcone et al., 1975).

Limitations of space compel us to omit many significant details of the schizophrenic process. The reader interested in Sullivan's ideas about schizophrenia may find them chiefly in *Conceptions of Modern Psychiatry*, *The Interpersonal Theory of Psychiatry* and *Clinical Studies in Psychiatry* (Sullivan 1953, 1956).

REFERENCES

American Psychiatric Association, Task Force on Nomenclature and Statistics. DSM III—Diagnostic and Statistical Manual of Mental Disorders 3rd ed., Washington, D.C., AMA, 1980.

Arieti, S. *Interpretation of Schizophrenia* 2nd ed.. Basic Books, New York, 1974.

Bemporad, Jr. Perceptual disorders in schizophrenia. *Am. J. Psychiat.* 1967; 123: 971–975.

Berger, P.L. and Luckman, T. *The Social Construction of Reality.* Doubleday, New York, 1966.

Bleuler, E. Autistic thinking. *Am. J. Insanity* 1913; 69: 873.

Bleuler, E. *Dementia Praecox on the Group of Schizophrenia* (trans. by Zinkin, J., 1911, from German). Internation Universities Press, New York, 1950.

Bowers, M.B., Jr. *Retreat from Sanity —The Structure of Emerging Psychosis.* Penguin Books, New York, 1974.

Carpenter, W.T., Jr. *Prognosis in Schizophrenia Prediction and Outcome.* CME series. Ledorle, University of Maryland, 1977.

Coleman, J.C. *Abnormal Psychology and Modern Life* 4th ed.. Scott, Foresman and Co., New York, 1972.

Ellenberger, H.E. *The Discovery of the Unconscious.* Basic Books, New York, 1970, pp. 531–532.

Hartman, E. Sleep, in Nicholi, A.M., Jr. ed.. *The Harvard Guide to Modern Psychiatry.* Belknap Press, Cambridge, 1975.

Havens, L.L. *Approaches to the Mind.* Little, Brown and Co., Boston, 1973.

Sullivan, H.S. *Conceptions of Modern Psychiatry.* W.W. Norton, New York, 1953.

Sullivan, H.S. *The Interpersonal Theory of Psychiatry.* W.W. Norton, New York, 1953.

Sullivan, H.S. *Clinical Studies in Psychiatry.* W.W. Norton, New York, 1956.

Van Praag, H.M. About the impossible concept of schizophrenia. *Comp. Psychiat.* 1976; 17: 481–497.

Zarcone, V., Jr., Azumi, K.K., et al. REM phase deprivation and schizophrenia II. *Arch. Gen. Psychiat.* 1975; 32: 1431–1436.

8

The Manic-Depressive Psychosis

Sullivan asserted that, in some unclear fashion, depression is closely related to manic and hypomanic states. In these states, there is said to be a great outburst of fleeting impulses to integrate situations with others, and a great variety of abbreviated integrations. There is a great volubility, which usually has low communicative value, because there is also great distractability of attention and "flight of ideas." The manic or hypomanic person manifests a corresponding acceleration of physiological processes and a remarkable increase in bodily movements. "The manic person is preoccupied with nothing; it is as if his attention shifted as frequently as possible, without rhyme or reason excepting the availability of some new distraction" (Sullivan, 1953).

Sullivan said that he had little to offer by way of theoretic importance on the manic depressive psychosis (See American Psychiatric Association, 1980). He varied between two notions about it. According to one, the central theme of manic excitement, that is, "the distractability, the flight of ideas," is to be considered as strongly conditioned by life situations. Sullivan's other notion is that manic-depressive states are to be regarded as primarily a disturbance of metabolism or "something of that kind." He believed that there has to be some disturbance of the commonplace biophysico-chemical existence of the person in order for him to maintain the enormous expenditure of energy, for this would ordinarily reduce one to utter inactivity before long.

The field of affective disorders has been radically altered since Sullivan lived and lectured. It is not our intention to cover the development of this specific field in this book. A thorough discussion of the affective disorders in view of the recent advances in the field can be found in Freedman et al. (1980); Nicholi (1978); and Usdin (1977).

Research on the metabolism of biogenic amines in depressive and manic patients has uncovered many clues to the biochemical pathophysiology of affective disorders. The introduction of drugs, effective in the treatment of depressions (mono amino oxidase inhibitors, antidepressants, and tricyclic antidepressants) and manias (lithium salts) has had a major impact on clinical psychiatry and the biological research in the field. Two main biochemical systems (involving norepinephrine and serotonin) are of major interest to the investigators in the field (Sourkes, 1977; Zarcone et al., 1977). Other complex systems and neurotransmitters (like acetylcholine) seem to play also an important role in affective disorders (Cazzoll et al., 1978) and endocrine changes are usually found (Rubin and Kendler, 1977). The biochemical, genetic-familial, life events, environmental stresses and the personality as well as psychodynamic factors have been all shown to contribute to the development of manic depressive disorder (Klerman, 1978), and influenced the current classification of affective disorders as represented in the Diagnostic and Statistical Manual of Mental Disorders III (American Psychiatric Association, 1980).

The element of duration in relation to onset baffled Sullivan. He said that people can go into a manic state quite swiftly. Manic states grow by accretion in such a fashion that the change is from a barely perceptible beginning to a very perceptible condition.

> Thus the appearance of the excitement is not *sudden*, even though the excitement may mount very rapidly in the course of, say, 24 hours, with a person passing from an irritable, uncomfortable type of active existence to a psychotic excitement. In other words, it is difficult to say just when a person becomes excited (Sullivan, 1956).

The growth of excitement by accretion was allegedly part of the argument in favor of the idea that somatological factors are causally connected with the manic-depressive psychosis. Sullivan thought that one will find depression deepens in much the same way if one looks at the other side of the manic-depressive picture. However, that is not as easy to detect, since the person's depression impresses "the innocent bystander" as being related to a particular event, perhaps deepening thereafter.

There is said to be a great deal of obvious hostility in quite a number of cases of manic excitement. In other cases, the pattern of activity reveals the hostility. For example, Sullivan gave a brief account of "the most amiable manic" he had ever known, who happened to be a wealthy woman (1956). "Her family," he said, "would know she had an attack when she would drive down the main street at 60 miles an hour and wave to the traffic cop, who was so flabbergasted that he didn't even whistle at her." When this sort of thing happened her family knew "she was well up, and it was time for the mental hospital." She is said to have been an amazingly genial woman who could crack jokes by the hour. But, when she was "up," excited, she violated all sorts of standards and rules—"although she did it gaily."

As previously mentioned, there are patients in the manic state whose hostility shows quite frankly. Sullivan mentioned another patient whom he had seen in a mental hospital. This patient, at the height of his excitement, could not resist the impulse to strike the night supervisor, who was a man twice his age, and generally a pretty kindly person. "This," Sullivan asserted, "was a clear instance of the ungovernable necessity for destructiveness and injury to others which appears in some patients at the height of their excitement and which is, I believe, part of the picture, even if masked" (Sullivan, 1956). It is noteworthy that lithium—the most important and potent chemical used today in the treatment of mania, can have an inhibitory effect on impulsive aggressive behavior not associated with psychosis (Sheard et al., 1976). Moreover, aggressive behavior is included as an official characteristic of Manic states in the recent DSM III (American Psychiatric Association, 1980).

Much less strikingly consistent, Sullivan said, is the discharge of other motivational systems. There are, he maintained, people who have a great expansion of their lust and engage in extremely manic sexual relations in the state of excitement. There are still others who, only after they have become impotent, become excited. While lust may color their thoughts, it does not lead to genital activity. Sometimes, motivational sets which have only appeared obscurely during the patient's waking hours manifest themselves with rather startling clarity in excitement. The "overloading" of the sublimation of some powerful drive often reveals the thing that has been sublimated after excitement. Imagine a person who has not seemed to noticeably deviate from a heterosexual *modus vivendi*. Assume, further, that fairly early in life he had slight warnings that he could not form any real attachment to a woman. This was indicated by an undue interest in members of his own sex. But the barrier to relationships of any consequence with women has been "gathered into" a sublimatory way of life. If lust is the drive that has been sublimated, Sullivan expected that such a person will "blow up" into an excitement. It may be that this person will engage in his first homosexual affair during the excitement.

MANIC EXCITEMENT AND SCHIZOPHRENIC EXCITEMENT

The picture one encounters in manic excitement is said to be the classic one or a slight variation of it. According to the classic formulation, the patient is both enormously energetic and extravagantly euphoric. As previously mentioned, physical activity is outstanding, although it has one "queer" characteristic. Sullivan meant that the large joint movements are facilitated, so that the elbow may be moved when one would ordinarily move the wrist, or the shoulder may be moved when one would ordinarily move the elbow. The content ("meaning"), Sullivan thought, is best apprehended as a manifestation of a constant necessity to have something going on in consciousness, but, since whatever is going on seems to get troublesome almost at once, there is a necessity to keep moving, as it were, from one thing to something else. Part of the physical activity may be that of the eyes literally darting around looking for things for the person to talk about.

> The most amazing ingenuity is shown in maintaining this distractability, such as using clang associations to something heard in the environment; almost anything that can come in by any of the sensory channels is grist for the mill (Sullivan, 1956).

Sullivan repeatedly had the inescapable impression that the hypomanic keeps busy by moving from one thing to another, lest he experience a drop in euphoria.

At one time it was believed that manic excitement ensued upon the collapse of the sublimatory organization, constituting the start of a manic-depressive history, as in schizophrenia. During the later part of his career, Sullivan thought that this idea is improbable and that, although the excitement of a schizoprhenic breakdown can at first be typically manic, it becomes less so in the course of time and winds up as a definite schizophrenic illness.

Sullivan arrived at the same conclusion with regard to excitement in the young, that is, in the periods of middle and late adolescence. In his long experience, he said, excitements have never initiated a manic-depressive history but, instead, had initiated schizophrenia. He had observed several youngsters brought into the hospital, where he had once worked, in a state of manic excitement. When they were beginning to quiet down, he heard them express "very foggy concepts" which he surmised represented more or less unusual implicit operations. Nevertheless, they were soon discharged from the hospital as social recoveries (wherein it was assumed they were so mentally disordered that they had required hospitalization and care, and were now free from any signs or symptoms of the disorder) or as being improved. They were then sent home and perhaps sent back to school, etc. Possibly a year later, Sullivan said, they were brought back to the hospital in an excited state. This time, he said, no one could mistake their excited states as those of the manic-depressive. These states were now *"definitely catatonic excitements."* The sublimatory organization which had collapsed had involved such things as hatred and fear of a parent (Sullivan, 1956).

THE ALTERNATION OF MANIC AND DEPRESSED STATES AND THE CLASSIFICATION OF THE AFFECTIVE DISORDERS

Kraepelin described manic-depressive psychosis as a mental state characterized by recurrent depressions and excitements or recurrent depressions or recurrent excitements. Thus, both phases may appear in cycles or only one phase may recur at more or less regular intervals. In some cases, the spacing of attacks is said to be rather remarkably regular, although in others, the regularity "just is not there." In the latter instances, such people may have suffered fairly difficult manic-depressive illnesses. Yet, they do not suffer another attack "until something remotely like an excuse comes along." After they recover from that, they may have another attack soon afterwards or they may never have another attack that is subject to observation.

An extensive and expensive effort is being made to learn more about the affective disorders in a five-year collaborative project now in progress under the National Institute of Mental Health (NIMH) auspices. The goals of this project are to determine the usefulness and validity of various ways of classifying affective disorders. During an early pilot phase of the project, a set of diagnostic criteria was developed and tested, which include an exhaustive structured interview and rating scale (Schedule for Affective Disorders and Schizophrenia—SADS). An operational set of criteria for Major Psychiatric Disorders (Research Diagnostic Criteria—RAD), which provided the format for the American Psychiatric Association's third Diagnostic and Statistical Manual (DSM III), is also used. The cyclicity and regularity of the manic-depressive episodes is expressed clearly in the recently published DSM III (American Psychiatric Association, 1980) and, although this study faces some strategical problems, including reliability, subclassifications (bipolar I, II, endogenous versus reactive, etc.), the presence or absence of precipitating events and others, the study's advantage is in its large 'n' including patients from all over the United States, which promises generalizability. It is hoped that major questions of classification of the affective disorders will be resolved in the near future (Gonzalez, 1980).

Depressed States

Sullivan (1953) taught that depression is only superficially related to grief and mourning. Depression is said to be chiefly a destructive dynamism which "cuts off" impulses to integrate situations, and such situations are extremely stereotyped. The person who suffers a deep depression is preoccupied with a circle of ideas about evil, hopelessness, destruction and damnation.

However, in *Clinical Studies in Psychiatry*, Sullivan (1953) claimed that the depression in the manic-depressive psychosis is a preoccupation of consciousness with a very restricted progression of grief-provoking ideas. It is also characterized, he said, by a more or less striking reduction of activity, relatively frequently in the large movements of the skeletal muscles. However, the slowing up is not restricted to the skeletal muscles anymore than the speeding up is confined to the skeletal muscles in the manic. In both phases, manic and depressive, there is a corresponding change in the activity of the visceral musculature. In general, in depressed states there is a change in the individual's physiology such that vital processes are slowed down. (This seems to be confirmed today. See previous reports on this issue in this chapter.)

The grief-provoking ideas of the depressive state are said to be viewed by the patient as an entirely adequate mental state in so far as he is alert enough to have an opinion about them. But, if the psychiatrist attempts to explore what any of these could mean, or what is wrong with them, he encounters irritation or anger, provided the patient is sufficiently "reactive." This is what Sullivan found in his limited experience with manic-depressives.

But, he also surmised that other people are meant to suffer from the patient's depression. Sometimes, the actions of the depressed person are clearly punitive. Occasionally, when it becomes evident that there is nobody who would suffer from them, the troublesome performances of a depressed patient disappear. Sullivan claimed,

> Even though this cannot be observed in each case, I find it very easy to presume that there is something other than loving kindness in the interpersonal relations of the depressed patient, particularly in the light of the quite impressive tendency toward hostility and convention-breaking found in the manic (Sullivan, 1956).

At times, a depressed spouse who becomes separated or divorced would no longer show depressive symptoms, but will easily display the aggression that Sullivan suspected.

PSYCHOGENESIS OF THE MANIC-DEPRESSIVE PSYCHOSIS

Sullivan flatly stated that the manic-depressive remained a mystery to him. As some of Sullivan's more friendly colleagues who are still alive today can testify, Sullivan's knowledge of people covered an extraordinarily broad range. In any event, he stated that he was unable to explain the psychogenesis of the manic-depressive psychosis. He was unable to get any real clues about it. However, he did say that his ability to work with people who suffer this psychosis was rather limited. Some of his former students and colleagues (Robert A. Cohen, Mabel Blake Cohen, Frieda Fromm-Reichman, etc.) carried out an intensive investigation of 12 manic-depressive patients and made certain important discoveries with regard to their interpersonal relations. They also attempted to relate them to the reported early life history of these patients (Cohen, 1980).

Ronald R. Fieve, one of the earliest psychiatrists to use lithium carbonate as a prophylaxis for manic-depressive disease, lends support to Sullivan's comments on the treatment of the manic-depressive patient with a psychogenetic (what can be referred to as a "psychoanalytic") approach. Fieve (1975) recalls his own training as a psychoanalyst and his frustrations in attempting to help patients with depression or manic-depressive illness with the analytic approach. He does discount "the talking cure" as appropriate treatment for some distressed persons, but notes that many individuals with symptoms responsive to pharmacotherapy no longer desire analysis or psychotherapy once they have been helped with drugs.

COHEN'S RESUME OF THE 12 PATIENTS

The following is a partial summary of what Cohen and his associates (1980) discovered: The patients were highly dependent on the esteem and approval of others. It was found that, in correlation with this dependency, they held values which were both conventional and changeable in conformity with what they perceived to be those of their group.

> They were unusually competitive and almost childish in their envy of others; the defense of denial was often employed, and associated with this was an insensitivity to the feelings of others and to their own motivations.

In exchange for approval of the person on whom they were dependent, they appeared to have abandoned any desire to achieve maturity and self-sufficiency. They tried to gain approval by doing whatever they believed that person on whom they were dependent wanted them to do. They were, nevertheless, intensely envious and competitive. Hence, they had become entrapped in a wretched dilemma.

> Their own pervasive envy of others led them to fear becoming themselves objects of envy by others. Consequently, they also feared success in achieving the dependent aims they persistently sought.

Cohen and his associates (See Cohen, et al., 1980) found that the family histories of the 12 manic-depressive patients were: (1) isolation of the family from the social environment by some factor such as economic, religious, or racial difference; (2) parental awareness of this difference and extraordinary efforts to maintain or raise family status by strict conformity to accept values; (3) parental manipulation of the children to gain the desired status, with the ultimate effect that the patient came to value himself in proportion to his conformity to these values; (4) continued emphasis in the family on the absolute need for conventional success, with resulting feelings of high competitiveness with and envy of others; (5) in most intensively studied cases, greater aggressiveness, ambition, and rigidity in the mother than in the father, who was blamed for the sad family state from which the patient was the potential rescuer; and (6) notable inconsistencies in discipline, in which the child was at times punished for behavior that at other times brought no reaction.

There have been several attempts by different psychoanalysts to understand the psychoanalytic roots of manic-depressive disorder which—we consider to be unsuccessful and hence, do not intend to discuss. The reader is referred to Jacobson (1971).

REFERENCES

American Psychiatric Association, Task Force on Nomenclature and Statistics. DSM III — Diagnostic and Statistical Manual of Mental Disorders 3rd ed.. Washington, D.C., AMA, 1980.

Cazzoll, B.J., Greden, J.F., Rubin, R.T., Haskett, R., Feinberg, M., and Schteingort, D. Neurotransmitter mechanism of neuroendocrine disturbances in depression. *Acta. Endocrinol.* Suppl., Copenhagen, 1978; 89:14.

Cohen, R.A. Manic-Depressive Reactions, in Freedman, A.M., Kaplan, H.I., and Sadock, B.J. eds.. *Comprehensive Textbook of Psychiatry III*. Williams and Wilkins, Baltimore/London, 1980. Originally published in *Psychiatry*, 1954.

Fieve, R.R. *Moodswing*. William Morrow, New York, 1975.

Freedman, A.M., Kaplan, H.I., Sadock, B.J. eds.. *Comprehensive Textbook of Psychiatry III*. Williams and Wilkins, Baltimore/London, 1980.

Gonzalez, E.R. Can depression be categorized? *JAMA* 1980; 18; 243: (15) 1505–08.

Jacobson, E. *Depression*. International Universities Press, New York, 1971.

Klerman, G.L. Affective disorders, in Nicholi, A.M., Jr. ed.. *The Harvard Guide to Modern Psychiatry*. Belknap Press, Cambridge, 1978.

Nicholi, A.M., Jr. ed.. *The Harvard Guide to Modern Psychiatry*. Belknap Press, Cambridge, 1978.

Rubin, R.T., and Kendler, K.S. Psychoneuroendocrinology: Fundamental Concepts and Correlates in Depression, in Usdin, G. ed.. *Depression*. Brunner Mazel, New York, 1977.

Sheard, M.H., Mazini, J.L., Bridges, C.I., and Wagner, E. Effect of lithium on impulsive aggressive behavior in man. *Am. J. Psychiat.* 1976; 133: 1409–1413.

Sourkes, T.L. Biochemistry of mental depression. *Can. Psychiat. Assoc. J.* 1977; 22: 467–481.

Sullivan, H.S. *Conceptions of Modern Psychiatry.* W.W. Norton, New York, 1953.

Sullivan, H.S. *Clinical Studies in Psychiatry.* W.W. Norton, New York, 1956.

Usdin, G. ed.. *Depression.* Brunner Mazel, New York, 1977.

Zarcone, V.P., Jr., Berger, P.A., Keith, H., Brodie, H., Sack, R., and Barchas, J.D. Indoleamine hypothesis of depression: Overview and pilot study. *Dis. Nerv. Sys.* 1977; 36: 646–653.

9

The Psychiatric Interview

Sullivan has called his therapeutic procedures "participant observation." Unfortunately, most psychiatrists have been unable to "explain" this, even when they have an intuitive grasp of its meaning. In order to understand the meaning of participation one must have an understanding of transaction, which is radically different from interaction, whose meaning in psychiatry is quite imprecise. Dewey and Bentley (1949) will be paraphrased in order to clarify some of the following conceptions.

In the history of Western thought, three fundamental assumptions have reigned. Each of these originated at a given time in a given social milieu. The first key concept is self-action. Dewey and Bentley (1949) have characterized it as follows: the "pre-scientific presentation in terms of presumptively independent 'actions,' 'souls,' 'minds,' (as in John Locke), 'selves,' 'powers,' or 'forces,' taken as activating events." Thus, according o this notion, things and persons are viewed as acting under their powers. Two good examples of this view are the theories of St. Augustine and Sigmund Freud, the former attributing remarkable powers to the Soul, and the latter to the Libido and the Thanatos.

Galileo and Newton introduced the notion of interaction. But, note that the prefix "inter" has two sets of applications (See the Oxford English Dictionary). One is for "between," "in-between," or "between the parts of." The other is for "mutually," "reciprocally." The result of this shifting use of the prefix as it enters philosophy, logic, and psychology, no matter how inadvertently, is ambiguity and undependability (Dewey and Bentley, 1949). This ambiguity has left most psychiatrists confused when they encounter Sullivan's use of transaction, and yet it would seem Sullivan made use of transaction perfectly clear in his *Conceptions of Modern Psychiatry* (1953) which is discussed at the beginning of chapter Two.

Dewey and Bentley went on to write:

It is here proposed to eliminate ambiguity by confining the prefix *inter* to cases in which "in-between" is dominant and to employ the prefix *trans* where the mutual and reciprocal are intended, and that is what psychiatrists usually mean when they talk or write about "interaction," though they are not always consistent — beause they can't be. Their subject matter compels them toward "mutuality and reciprocity" — toward transaction.

That is the other meaning of "inter." Summarily, Sullivan abandoned the familiar use of interaction for transaction. What then is transaction? Without going into details, it was Maxwell (1949) (with the work of Faraday before him) who mathematically formulated the notion of a "field." Thus, he wrote:

> Physical science, which up to the end of the eighteenth century has been fully occupied in forming a conception of natural phenomena as a result of forces acting between one body and another, has now fairly entered the next stage of progress — that in which the energy of a material system is conceived as determined by the *configuration*, motion, and force are generalized to the utmost extent warranted by their physical definitions.

In his book, *Matter and Motion*, Maxwell (1949) employed the term transaction in describing events. Einstein and Infeld (1938) have declared that, in Maxwell's view, there are no material actors. Summarily, there are three levels of organization and presentation of inquire: self-action, interaction, and transaction.

In harmony with Sullivan's formulation of transaction, traditional notions of "inner forces," "drives," or whatever, have two widely separated aspects. Whatever occurs beneath the skin is not self-contained or isolated. Inner processes (traditionally called the "subjective" side of man) and outer, overt processes (traditionally called the "behavioral" side of man) are part of one comprehensive configuration. The simplest illustration (apart from Sullivan's discussion of the living cell in the uterus, which follows the principle of transaction before and after birth and thenceforward through life) one can think of is breathing. It is not an affair of the lungs alone. In this connection, the experience of drowning is most persuasive. The lungs, physically isolated within the body, taken by themselves, do not "explain" breathing. Given a functioning organism, the surrounding atmosphere is as much a part of the breathing cycle as are the lungs and attendant organs. Transaction reigns in all human life.

Hence, for Sullivan, the study of interpersonal relations is always a study of a situation or configuration. The data of psychiatry arise in *participant observation* due to a given configuration. There is no such thing as an isolated person, for interpersonal relations include the "symbolic" or a "blend" of the real and the symbolic. This in no way denies various organic processes. They form the "substrate" of human life. (Even the "organic" psychoses have an interpersonal aspect.) The interview is a situation of primary *vocal* communication on a "progressively unfolding expert-client basis for the purpose of *elucidating patterns of living* of the subject person (patient or client) (1956). These patterns which the client experiences are especially valuable. In the interview, both the assets and the liabilities of the patient must be assessed. Sullivan could be very scornful of psychiatrists who ignored or slighted the assets of the client. This kind of "therapy" Sullivan thought could be thoroughly destructive.

Sullivan thought that interpersonal situations imply something more than the presence of two people somewhere. The two people are *involved* with each other—they are integrated. An interpersonal situation is brought into being by, held together by, and the course of their events or processes are to a certain extent determined by, something in the two people which is *reciprocal*, the manifestations of which coincide approximately in time. "Thus one may say that the interview situation, or series of situations, is integrated by *coincident reciprocal motivation* of interviewee (or client) and interviewer (the therapist)" (Sullivan, 1956).

The therapist or interviewer has the task of so influencing the interview situation that the closely observed course of his participation will reveal the major handicaps and major advantages in living which are relatively durable characteristics of the interviewee (Sullivan, 1954). for example, the "obsessional personality" will, day in and day out, try to control every interpersonal situation he has become involved in. A simple illustration is stuttering. And yet, the underlying is not so much control but to *ward off anxiety* by his various security operations. In general, he is painfully vulnerable to the slings, arrows, and slights of his wife or girl friend.

The following gives a very lucid account of the logic of interviewing:

It is the interpersonal events and the pattern of their course which generate the data of the interview; that is, the interviewer experiences the ways in which the interpersonal events follow each other, what seeming relationships they have to one another, what striking inconsistencies occur, and so on. Thus the data of the interview may come, not so much from the answers to questions, but from the timing and stress of what was said, the slight misunderstandings here and there, the occasions when the interviewee got off the subject, perhaps volunteering very important facts which had not been asked for, and so on. And so as the interviewer grows more skillful, he realizes with increasing clarity that what he must do is watch the course of events and observe how they, as a pattern of progression, give rise to a very wide field of data about the other person with whom he is concerned ("integrated"). His use of this data, and his skill in drawing inferences from it, will grow with experience. Yet, until he has the information to be gained from this kind of participant observation, he has nothing with which to begin; and it cannot be obtained by the charmingly simple procedure of sitting at a desk and, with a feeling of utterly detached isolation from the person out in front, shooting questions at him, and perhaps checking his answers on a form (Sullivan, 1956).

In order to circumvent this kind of futile "analysis," Sullivan formulated four stages in the organization of the interview. All psychiatric data are said to arise from participation in the situation that is observed-participant observation. One must be alert to the possibilities of the immediate future of the relationship in which one is involved. Therefore, Sullivan taught that the psychiatrist, in so far as it is possible, concentrates his attention on the processes going on between himself and the other person, or involving himself and the other person, and not on something as remote as "What is this patient of mine doing and saying…"

STAGES OF THE INTERVIEW

There are four stages: (1) The Formal Inception; (2) The Reconnaissance; (3) The Detailed Interview; (4) The Termination of the Interview (Sullivan, 1956).

The Formal Inception

First, one must consider the actual "physical" encounter with the interviewee or client. He may be a stranger or an old friend who gradually in the course of conversation "converts himself" into a client. Sullivan claimed that the way in which the client is received can greatly accelerate the achievement of the desired result, or it can make the result practically unattainable.

> From the moment that the interviewer and the interviewee first see each other, very important aspects of the psychiatric interview are in progress. And from this moment, the interviewer must realize that his own convenience, his own past malfeasances, and so on, are not anywhere near as important as the assumption that here is someone to be treated with respectful seriousness because he wants to be benefited or at least can be benefited (Sullivan, 1954).

This implies that the psychiatrist never greets his patient with a lot of social hokum — quite in contrast to the conventional smiles, handshakes, embraces, etc., of many people in the great world in which the client customarily lives. Patients don't like to be treated as statistical instances of how the doctor or nurse greets people when they arrive at the office.

So, when a prospective patient arrived at Sullivan's door, the latter did *not* try to show great welcome. Sullivan did try to show that the patient was expected, asking the name of the person who recommended him and thus relieving the patient of any morbid anxiety as to whether he came on the wrong day, or to the wrong place, etc. Sullivan would then invite him in. He would take a good look at the patient while he was at the door, but after that he would not stare at him. When he was in the office, the interviewer would indicate where the former should sit and so relieve him of any confusion about this.

Next, Sullivan would tell the patient what he had learned about him with regard to why he came. When the client or patient telephoned to make an appointment, Sullivan might say, "I gathered from our conversation over the phone that you have a problem of such-and-such a nature," using a slightly rising inflection and so putting a little question mark at the end. If Sullivan knew why the patient was there because another doctor had sent him, or the chief of the hospital division, or someone else, he would say, "I gather it is for such-and-such reasons," again in a slightly questioning tone. In this superficially simple manner, Sullivan has already demonstrated to the patient that he had paid attention to what little data had been presented to him, including what was said over the phone. So, from the very beginning, Sullivan has given the patient a chance to react, and a magnificent opportunity to revise the information elicited. And so, the patient may say "Yes, that's right Doctor, and it's a great problem" or, instead, "What? Why I never dreamed of it. How is it possible for you to have such a misunderstanding?" With his usual skill Sullivan would reply, "Well now, tell me what really *is* the case." And then the patient may begin to tell him—although it is very unlikely that he knows what really is the case. Actually, as soon as Sullivan subtly starts to probe, he may receive any one of a host of responses—but that is not significant for our account in the present context. At this early stage, Sullivan is likely to tread softly with a disturbed patient because he does not yet know what really "ails the patient." And at this stage it would be, or could be, dangerous to therapeutic progress.

At this first stage, the psychiatrist should have "some idea" of how he affects the stranger and how he facilitates or retards certain things that the stranger may have thought of doing. The psychiatrist, according to Sullivan, should also have learned what sorts of immediate impressions he himself obtains from the appearance, initial movements, and vocal behavior of another (the client). He should note that in such a relationship, what one hears first from the other person, no matter "how free and easy," or how conventional, represents that person's repertoire of operations to be addressed to a complete stranger. The psychiatrist, at this early phase has the definite necessity of having some idea of how the patient's operations affect him, the interviewer. Also, the psychiatrist must be scrupulously careful not to do anything that is exterior to his consciousness which will greatly handicap the development of the interview situation, or which will direct the development of the interview in an unnecessarily obscure way. One must know what one is doing and how it affects the patient. Thus, one must be careful not to unwittingly prohibit, forbid, or "shoo" the patient away from a particular type of data. Because, for example, at this stage, the client may be made very anxious. Sullivan was very caustic about therapists who don't know how to circumvent very disturbing potential data, until the time is ripe, usually during the *Detailed Interview*.

During the Inception, Sullivan was keenly aware that during this phase the doctor cannot *know* what is going on in the patient's mind. At best, he can have a useful surmise of *alternate* probabilities largely derived from his experiences with other patients. The best he can do is keep two probabilities in mind. As he explores or tests them, the probability of one declines, while the other increases. In this fashion, the interviewer gradually progresses toward reasonable accuracy. This limitation will not be employed during later phases of the interview.

Finally, Sullivan held that the interviewer should be alert to, so that he can correctly recall, all that he has said and done in the formal inception of each interview, so that he can learn to do better. He must be able to recall a course of events correctly—the timing of movement, what preceded what, what followed what, etc. In other words, not only communication by speech, but communication by gesture, broadly conceived, an interchange by expressive movement other than speech—the beginning of working hypotheses about the person.

The Reconnaissance

In this, the second stage Sullivan (1956) would set out to obtain a rough social sketch of the patient, which is brief, and not an extended history.

Customarily, Sullivan began this stage by saying, "Now tell me how old are you? Where were you born? Are your mother and father living?" If one or both parents are dead, he would ask, "When did they die and of what?" Suppose the patient doesn't know what his father, for example, died of; this "information" may lead to the discovery that the father hasn't lived in the home for the past 20 years, and that while the patient is pretty sure his father is dead, he doesn't know any of the circumstances. These are important data. Next, the interviewer asks how many siblings there are, including any who died. This inquiry may be significant if a sibling died during the memory span of the patient. Also, it is important to note those siblings who died before the patient can remember, because they might have been of particular significance to his parents and thus have a considerable effect on him. The interviewer would ask the place of the patient in the time-order of siblings. Then comes the question of who, besides the parents, was chronically or frequently in the home during the patient's first seven years; an uncle, an aunt, a grandmother, for example. The presence of the relative may leave a quite permanent influence. The reason is that his grandmother may have been the only bright spot in the patient's home during the first seven years of his life and he may be glad to be reminded of her. It may be that she shielded him, as best as she could, from bodily harm, or an unremitting repertory of derogatory remarks, daily.

Then would come questions about the father. While many variants, such as the geographical, the economic, etc., have played a role in the life history of the father, it is much more illuminating to learn what sort of person the father was, if it is possible.

But, before that, the interviewer would ask who in the family supported it. At the present time, one can fairly easily understand why Sullivan inquired about any marked economic disturbances that may have occurred, either for general or specific reasons, because they have very marked effects on the course of personality development. Long ago, Sullivan thought that parents almost always aim their children at something which they either seek or avoid at all costs. Hence, big economic changes may lead to a tragic, heartbreaking revision of the parental ambitions, with accompanying, corresponding effects on the children's ambitions and goals — an outcome which may have left permanent marks on the patient's future. When there are changes, the interviewer should try to discover at approximately what age they occurred in the interviewee's life. It is almost axiomatic that the earlier a child suffers psychological damage, the more profound and long lasting the consequences tend to be. For that and other reasons, Sullivan would try to discover how early these changes occurred: for example, before the patient was eight. In this instance, the parents, by their efforts and utterances, may have greatly influenced the child, that is, in order to direct his life. On the other hand, if the patient was 18–21 years old when the changes occurred, they may affect or destroy his chances to enter a university, or pursue the professions of medicine or law. Or, if he has been graduated and completed his education, these changes probably have not made very much difference, except in so far as he has other people dependent on him.

When Sullivan had gathered all this information and more, he became curious about the father in regard to what sort of person the patient was. This kind of questioning leads people to become anything from vocal to helpless. Should the patient become helpless in such context, Sullivan would try to give him a helping hand. So, the interviewer would ask with regard to the father, "Well, how was he regarded in the community?" If the patient still remained helpless and inarticulate in the face of such questioning, Sullivan might ask about the pastor of the church, the family doctor, the druggist, the grocer and so on, "What would they have said of the father offhand?"

After Sullivan had obtained some idea of what sort of person the patient's father was, he would become "curious" to learn whether his family was a happy one, and whether the parents were happily married. For reasons unstated, Sullivan would then want to know about the mother. Thus, while Sullivan would ask what sort of person the father was, he would ask the patient to *describe* his mother. Usually, the patient has an exceedingly vague notion of his mother. Next, Sullivan would ask what sort of people (previously mentioned) stayed around the house a great deal. This, he said, was or is usually such a relief to the patient after trying to describe his mother that "I often get quite an account of the third, the semiparent; and that semiparent may prove to be illuminating, if only in understanding the role that I may play later on in the relationship" (Sullivan, 1956).

Sullivan would then ask the patient to tell him something about his education. Following this, the interviewer will want to know about his occupational history which still includes big "factors" of the economic situation, along with the geographical opportunities, and so on, because they are much more illuminating as to the patient's ability to get on with people and to get somewhere in life. (Sullivan slighted education, since he thought educational factors are fortuitous indices of the combination of the foresight and blind ambition of the parents, wealthy relatives, and the patient.)

The occupational history informs the interviewer what the patient has done since leaving school. This is very important because the sicker people are, the more they omit from their occupational history. This omission is said to be a very important part of the psychiatric interview. Therefore, Sullivan would resort to the following stratagem: He would tell the patient what he had heard, and then inquire as to whether what he had been told was the whole story. He would say something like the following: "Well aside from those two jobs, you have had no other occupation?" It may turn out that the patient, in a given interview situation, may reveal that he has had 25 other jobs, although he hasn't held them for long. The point here is that the interviewer does not want to know particulars about the job. All he wants to know is what jobs the patient held, for how long, and where—so that he can get an idea of whether the person was advancing in his work; whether he was so driven by a need for money that he held a job only long enough to get one that paid more; whether he held each job long enough to know what the work was about and then took another one, "in a curiously thorough but superficially morbid pattern of learning something about life;" whether he quarreled with everyone that he ever tried to work with; and so forth. Sullivan did not want details, but he did want a sketch of the facts.

Then Sullivan became "curious" as to whether the patient was married, and if so, how long he had been married. He wanted to know if the patient was happily married. Should it turn out that it isn't a happy marriage, the patient usually pauses, and then replies "Yes." The interviewer may look at such a patient then and ask if there are any children. The former may go on to ask if it is the patient's first marriage. Quite often, the latter will say, "No, no, I was married before," making it sound as if the therapist should have known this—as if by psychiatric osmosis. Next, the interviewer wants to know about the first marriage. Was it the patient's first love? Should there be a little hesitancy, then there comes a related question. "Why did you marry?" Of course, the answers patients offer vary.

Thus, Sullivan would stop this line of questioning.

> Of the labels which the patient's neighbors and casual acquaintances attach to him, I have tried to pick up those that have some measure of probable significance for understanding what he does. He feels I know a great deal about him. . . . In a vague way, I do know a great deal, because from now on I just watch if the customary indices prove to be correct in his case, and wherein he is an exception to the probabilities which are implied in the semistatistical data of his past, his family position, and so on (Sullivan, 1956).

Sullivan thought it is necessary to leave the patient more or less in control of the topics. Things have to flow, for otherwise they are apt to be so disconnected that the interviewer does not quite know what he has learned. Thus, as the interviewee is more or less answering an orignial stream of questions, the interviewer has the opportunity, by alert listening and some observation, to pick up a great many clues for further exploration.

In the brief sketch already described, the interviewer utilizes as much as he can of the dubious (questionable), but still respectable generalizations that he has picked up in all his previous life and study, remembering, nevertheless, that those generalizations are statements of probability. This idea should not disturb the reader since all scientific statements are laws of probability, however mathematically rigorous they may be formulated. Even Newton's Second Law is a statement of probability and now appears to apply only within a limited cosmic sphere.

The Use of Free Association

During the reconnaissance, the interviewer may hear of some situation which occurred at some time in the patient's past which seems significant, but seems unclear. It is not accessible to the patient's consciousness, or as Freud might say, it has been "repressed." But Sullivan (1956) differed considerably from Freud's technique. The former would not urge the patient to say "every littlest thing that came to mind." Sullivan would say, "Well, I really wonder what might have been the case; tell me what comes to mind." Sullivan added that partly because of the pressure, partly because of the objectivity of the inquiry, and partly because the patient really is trying to get something out of his relationship with the interviewer's psychiatry, he often has a very surprising experience in discovering what comes to his mind. Sullivan would try to get the patient to talk more or less at random as things come to mind. As the latter begins to talk about what comes to his mind, his thoughts "will begin to circle" toward the answering of the question. Still, there will be a process of starting and stopping many a time before the very significant question is answered.

It is not until the patient has had a few examples of the fact that free association makes sense, that the psychiatrist can lay down injunctions about it to the point where he can advise the patient as to the inadvisability of his selecting what to report; that is, the psychiatrist can lay down useful injunctions as to what *not* to report at some given time. Thus, the patient begins to learn that the omitting of ideas because they seem irrelevant or immaterial may cause the therapeutic process to miscarry. (At this point, it is important to mention that anxiety is the greatest enemy of the free flow of thought.)

Summary of the Reconnaissance

Then there follows a summary of the reconnaissance in a brief manner (Sullivan, 1956). As he presents the summary, the interviewer should explain that he now wishes to tell the patient what has impressed him in the reconnaissance, and that he would like the patient to bear with him until he is through, so that he will be relatively interpreted. At the beginning of the summary, the psychiatrist should tell the patient that he will be asked to amend and correct those things which the psychiatrist has misunderstood, and to point out any important things which he has missed.

When the psychiatrist seriously attempts to summarize what has happened at the end of the reconnaissance, the patient will have an experience which in some ways is quite startling: Things that the patient has known all his life and which he has told the psychiatrist in the interviews will be reflected back to him in the summary in a newly meaningful fashion — in spite of what the psychiatrist thinks of as his own stupidities and forgetfulness. Thus to the extent that the summary represents a somewhat expert view of the data that the patient had accessible in his awareness and was moved to report in the interview, it will be a very uplifting experience to the patient—a very definite step in the patient's education as to how psychiatry works (Sullivan, 1956).

The patient may have caught on to the fact that, as the summary shows, he has unexpectedly revealed some of his conventional evasions and distortions.

A caveat is in order. Sullivan held that sometimes the problems in living which the psychiatrist encounters in the reconnaissance are so grave, so close to the structure of the most serious mental disorders, that it would be simply disastrous to toss them in the patient's face. But, Sullivan said one could refer to them obliquely without revealing anything directly about the patient's psychiatric difficulties.

As the reconnaissance comes to a close, the psychiatrist outlines what he sees as a major difficulty—or at least an alleged major problem. Hence, the doctor and the patient now have something to work on. Otherwise, without this statement, treatment is apt to be self-defeating. It may also happen that the patient decides he is getting nothing for his money and abandons therapy.

The Detailed Inquiry

The impressions one has gained during the first two stages are essentially hypotheses which must be "tested" (Sullivan, 1956). Hence, the detailed inquiry is a matter of improving on earlier approximations of understanding. During the detailed inquiry, a really revolutionary change in one's impressions may occur. From the beginning of the psychiatric interview, the therapist has to contend with the patient's anxiety—and sometimes his own. Patients are said to make statements that would have misled anyone who was paying attention only to what these statements *presumably* meant. For example, patients may say things which have so little to do with their "durable characteristics" that the psychiatrist finally realizes that one of the great difficulties in the interview is the patient's effort to suit him, to impress him. In other words, like other people, in and out of therapy, psychiatrists want to protect their self-esteem. Yet, the patient or client is completely unconscious of any intention of deceiving the psychiatrist or defeating him in his efforts to discover what is going on. Hence, the patient says things which are actually grossly misleading, and manages to say them as if they were absolute truths. History testifies to the fact that people have endured indescribable tortures in order to protect their self-esteem or self-respect.

As one might expect from a study of previous chapters, the interviewer does have to deal with anxiety almost eternally. The patient, as best he can, strives to maintain security or a feeling of well-being in any interpersonal situation unless some considerable merit is anticipated, which will make the suffering of anxiety worthwhile at least for a brief period. Attempts to ward off anxiety (a function of the self) are called *security operations*, not the *defense mechanisms* of Freud, although Kohut and other psychiatrists are striving to refine Freud's ideas.

The interviewer, therefore, has to deal with anxiety, which always—in contrast to fear—manifests in interpersonal relations. However, anxiety and fear may become intertwined. (In today's world, this seems to be almost commonplace.) Anxiety is dealt with in relation to others, for example, certain people who seem chronically irritable or angry are in fact, without realizing it, suffering from anxiety—and, therefore, is a work of exquisite refinement. This handling of anxiety with others is of crucial importance, at least until the patient sees a high probability that something useful is going to come of it. So, the psychiatrist must avoid any carelessness about provoking anxiety or any insensitivity to the manifestations of it. Failure in such instances tends to promote disaster (theorem of reciprocal emotion). Thus, if the therapist is treating an "obsessional" person and fails to tread lightly over his vulnerability, he may precipitate a schizophrenic episode.

Sullivan taught that anyone who proceeds without consideration for the disjunctive power of anxiety in human relations will never learn interviewing, that is, how to do successful therapy. Still, such a doctor may turn out to be an excellent physician in another specialty. If there is no consideration for anxiety, a true interview is said not to exist. The patient will try frantically to defend himself against some kind of devil (the therapist) who seems determined (as the patient experiences this dreadful situation) to set out to prove that the patient is a bad person. As Sullivan used to say in some of his lectures, psychotherapy is the hardest kind of work he knew.

In order to prove to his students the significance of anxiety operations, he proposed the following:

> What I have been saying about anxiety and security operations will become more meaningful if you will make a careful study of the next awkward situation that you get into with your boss, your husband or wife, or whatnot. Needless to say you will only be able to study this awkward situation retrospectively (Sullivan, 1956).

The "cause" of this sort of situation is anxiety, which distracts thought. Hence, the interviewer must learn to recognize the anxiety that underlies the situation-operation in the interviewee. Thus, the patient may seem to have gotten angry, forgetful, etc., even completely silent—unwitting disguises of his attempt to avoid a feeling that is painful and tends to make one feel helpless. The interviewer observes and studies such patterns of security operations. He tries to find out what underlies the sleeping behavior or the fireworks of anxious patients, and what changes in the interviewer's attitude, as reflected by the interviewee, have occurred. So, the skillful interviewer asks himself what the patient feels about the interviewer's attitude. And the latter usually has an idea of what may be the case in such a situation, a specultion based on his skill and experience.

GROSS IMPRESSIONS OF THE INTERVIEW SITUATION

Sullivan held that in order to observe change, it is necessary to have some point of departure; and for the detailed inquiry, that point of departure lies in those gross impressions obtained during the first two stages. The changes from those early gross impressions are said to be those which are observed during the later course of the interview as useful data as one proceeds.

First, the interviewer must ask whether the interview is hard going in terms of its efficiency. Or, is the interview rather "run-of-the-mill" and not in any way unusual? Then, he begins to analyze it from several points of view. First, he considers the *general alertness;* that is, does the patient show how keen he is and in how many areas. Also, the interviewee's *attention* to what is going on may vary greatly. Some people are very intent on what the therapist says, with the hope of getting something out of the interview. Other patients are *distracted* — either by the noises going on outside, or things going on in their own minds, all of which tend to impede the interview. Occasionally, a person's attitude may be described as *vague* — a very foggy and most casual attitude toward the interview and what he is trying to get at. So, the responses such patients produce seem at best to have a tenuous or nebulous relationship to what the other person has said. In addition to what the interviewer has learned, he develops an impression of the *intelligence* of the interviewee. But, one must guard against first impressions, which can be quite misleading. For example, the patient's tenuous command of the (English) language can be so poor that he may literally seem not to know the language. It may have happened that in his home, the patient's parents spoke Spanish or some other language. The parents may also neglect the patient in various ways. As he has grown up, he may have picked up enough of the language to drive a cab or even learn to handle complex machinery. Still, verbal dexterity is usually closely related to intelligence when there has been opportunity for the development of verbal skills. While language is a powerful instrument for learning truth, it can also be used—as in books—to disguise the truth. And it is often so used.

THE DEVELOPMENTAL HISTORY AS A FRAME OF REFERENCE

Sullivan held that throughout the development of the interview situation, however prolonged, the patient is manifesting efforts to avoid, minimize, and conceal signs of his anxiety from the interviewer and from his own locutions, behavior patterns, posturings, and pretensions. In this connection, consider the hysteric as he adopts various ruses.

A great deal has been said in earlier chapters about the self (also called the anti-anxiety system). This may be summed up in the following statement: "The interviewee's self-system is at all times, but in varying degrees, in opposition to achieving the purpose of the interview" (Sullivan, 1956).

Thus, the interviewer's skill is said to be concerned with circumventing the interviewee's security operations without increasing the scope or subtlety of these operations. It takes skill and experience in order to avoid calling out, provoking more security operations or more obscure and subtle ones.

Previously in the interview the psychiatrist will have gained a gross impression in three fields—"Is the patient being impressed with the therapist's expertness in interpersonal relations? Is the patient coming more and more to appreciate the therapist as an understanding person?" Consider a situation where a therapist is interviewing a 17-year old about the details of his sex life. The blunt questioner would produce so much anxiety, in all likelihood, that the adolescent would not even be able to stutter, and perhaps needless to say, would not produce anything useful. The third major question about the patient's impression of the interviewer relates to the patient's feeling about the simplicity of motivation in the therapist. Is the therapist solely interested in doing a competent job? Or to what extent does the patient seem to think that the therapist is motivated by ulterior purposes?

To the extent the patient's assessment is that the doctor has only benign motives, the serious work of the interview will be vastly expedited, and the difficulties of the patient's personality will be increasingly presented with a minimum of wear and tear on the doctor. Conversely, if the patient's assessment adds up to a belief that is not favorable, the data are presented in such a way as to make their interpretation more difficult. This means that the patient's ability to express himself is more restricted.

THE THEOREM OF RECIPROCAL EMOTION

This is one of Sullivan's (1953) central ideas. It reads as follows: Integration in an interpersonal situation is a process in which (1) complementary needs are resolved (or aggravated); (2) reciprocal patterns of activity are developed (or disintegrated); and (3) foresight of satisfaction (or rebuff) of similar needs is facilitated. Here are examples: (1) In interpersonal situations from early childhood onwards, because a person needs tenderness and frankness, anxiety aggravates the need for tenderness. (2) Reciprocal patterns of activity of various kinds are developed or disintegrated if disapproved by the significant other.

Thus there is or may be a need for reassurance. Sometimes the therapist responds indirectly by saying something which would sooner or later be seen as a favorable or hopeful outlook. Suppose the patient indicates a need for reassurance. If the therapist is clumsy or misses what the patient is trying to get at, he aggravates the patient's insecurity as well as the therapist's need to be reassured by the progress of the therapy. If the doctor needs reassurancce, he may communicate this by some activity which will "scare off, disparage or belittle the patient." Parenthetically, Sullivan was very severe with any of his students who acted sadistically with any of his patients. The result of the "sadistic," disparaging behavior of any interview is to aggravate his need for reassurance. In certain instances, the patient who has been disparaged will simply abandon therapy — at least with his present interviewer.

At times, when the patient will develop an alert foresight of the rebuff of his implied need for reassurance, he protects his self-esteem by various security operations. In such a case, the intelligent interviewer will try to observe what he is doing as best he can — or consult a more seasoned and secure therapist.

A SUGGESTED OUTLINE FOR OBTAINING DATA

According to Sullivan (1956), one of the first things which the interviewer might obtain information about is the patient's history of learning "toilet habits." The establishing of such patterns is usually begun, he asserted, before the end of infancy, and as a result, the patient's information about them is probably not formulated and would require months of investigation to bring any degree of certainty. But, one often may have picked up some clues about it.

Some of the really unfortunate people of the world are said to have been exposed to strict bowel training well before early childhood, and, as a result of their parents' abnormal interest (which is one aspect of the parents' personalities), have suffered rather grave difficulties in life thenceforth.

The parents' concern with toilet training is especially typical of the American middle classes. If Sullivan had been brought up in a peasant culture, he would have known that the parents in such a social milieu usually regard and treat the childrens' bowel functions casually and often with amusement. When the children get to be a little older, they troop off together out into the fields and make a sort of game of the elimination process.

Disorders of toilet habits may be obscurely reflected in personal cleanliness and in certain other things. The patient gives unusual attention to the chair on which he is about to sit, to the keeping of clothing from any casual contact with dust or dirt, to the careful preservation of creases in his trousers, etc. Sullivan tended to emphasize the *estimable qualities of the abnormality*. He would not want to frighten the interviewee away by too blunt reference to a careful thoughtfulness that he might consider peculiarly private or "strange." Parents who have produced tidy infants are said to be so proud of it that the children later hear about it —and the therapist in the course of his work gets to hear of it also.

This matter of personal cleanliness pertains to many things; not only to whether the patient is coarsely dirty but also to how carefully he has combed his hair, cleaned his fingernails, shaved, and all that sort of thing. It is fortunate that the therapist knows much more than what usually gets formulated, so that he can fairly easily get an impression of whether a person is clean, unkempt, or unclean; is tidy or very neat, etc. The point is, that if a person is ordinarily clean, and not unduly clean or unduly dirty, he is accepting the conventional norm. This suggests that the person has no "preternatural" interest in this field and thus leaves a little less work for the therapist to struggle with alone.

Sullivan also asserted that disorders in learning toilet habits may also be reflected, more subtly, in the patient's attitude toward certain words, which he regards as definitely offensive and does not use. Those are the words ordinarily considered "dirty." But, gradually, the psychiatrist may realize that a patient is a little restricted in his freedom to use such words as he knows.

Some other things that the interviewer may think of as connected to the period of toilet training are prolonged enuresis, habitual constipation, and recurrent diarrhea. The therapist can learn this information when it is faintly apropos and when the patient will probably not at all be offended and capable of giving the relevant information.

DISORDERS IN LEARNING SPEECH HABITS

In the more fortunate, the learning of speech habits is said to usually "collide" with the learning of toilet habits, although one or the other may take precedence for a little while. Next on the developmental scheme are *disorders* in learning speech (Sullivan, 1956). Such disorders may be manifested in faint suggestions of earlier trouble, such as hesitancy in speech, in oral over-activity (too much mouth activity), or in manneristic accompaniments of speech at times of stress. Sometimes, people employ very manneristic speech when they talk over the telephone.

All of these things are said to suggest that there may be great value in developing an interest in the distortions of personality occurring as far back as the learning of speech. This means that the signs that come to the interviewer's attention may all have some relationship to a history of disorders or deficiencies in speech habits, which the interviewer can discover by skillful, careful questioning. Any of the following may show up, such as delay in learning to speak, stuttering or lisping, peculiarities of vocabulary, and continued use of autistic or frankly neologistic terms.

If there is a delay in beginning to speak, it is usually not a manifestation of a morbid situation in which there is no sufficient need for learning speech behavior, and there is, in fact, a positive premium for *not* learning. Sullivan thought lisping may be partly organic; in any case it has a great social disadvantage and is, therefore, important to the patient's experience and behavior, however neurological or anatomical it may be. Sullivan thought that the more obscure distortions, such as peculiarities in speech or in vocabulary, are not disorders in acquiring speech behavior, but rather, defects in acquiring the knack of consensual validation, which is a form of verification, sometimes gross, as in the wave of a hand to a neighbor, and sometimes subtle. When one waves a hand to a neighbor it may simply mean "how are you?" The response usually consists of nodding, waving the hand, or simply smiling and nodding. In other words, one of those ways is, in effect, saying "I'm O.K." But, at its best, psychiatry in practice is often very subtle.

It is often said that people don't listen; and, if this is true, as it seems to be, it is serious enough. But, disorders in the realm of speech behavior are more widespread than most people realize. One may think that it is easy to believe what another person says, and vice versa. But, if one does not overlook negative instance, he would be greatly impressed with what idiosyncratic things people mean by words that they use to mean something different than they appear to. Sometimes, the patient's use of words is extraordinary; he appears to depend on a word to communicate something to the listener, which doesn't communicate this at all. In other words, he is still depending on a term used in everyday speech which doesn't communicate at all. Then, one realizes that the other person (or patient) is still quite autistic in his verbal thinking (as he often was in childhood), and that there has been a very serious impairment of this extremely important aspect of his socialization. This is said to reach its positively pathological state in the use of neologisms which have meaning and existence as "words" only in the mind of the user. Such use of neologisms indicates the presence of a serious problem.

In the catatonic schizophrenic state, autistic language often predominates, although in the patient's lucid moments he can use words intelligibly and clearly. Once, when giving a talk on Sullivan in a mental hospital, a visiting lecturer chatted briefly and lucidly with a person he thought was a visitor. He subsequently learned that the "attendant" was a schizophrenic patient. The patient talked and acted normally because the psychiatrist acted normally and spoke in a friendly fashion. Schizophrenic people, when they are not in the grip of the psychosis, are notoriously sensitive to the attitudes of other people.

The next topic to be discussed is games and partners in them. This pertains to the juvenile era. In general, during this era, the boy (and recently some girls) is inducted into games which represent a certain cooperation, a certain element of competition and often a very large element of compromise with compeers. There are some wonderful eccentricities that appear during the juvenile era, such as certain coteries Sullivan knew. These ladies and gentlemen would arise from bed in the late afternoon, dress rather carefully, "gather up their husbands or wives and proceed to the bridge club." According to Sullivan, there they would engage in an intensely concentrated performance, almost without speech or with highly formalized speech. They would spend a considerable number of hours pursuing this ritual, they then would "go out and retrieve their social remnant—by which I mean the mate—get something to eat, and go through a practically meaningless routine of life until the next meeting of the group (Sullivan, 1956). Sullivan added that this is not very much different from certain large prosperous communities which center more or less around a suburban country club. In those instances, all of life which is not involved in golf and the club is treated as a boring routine that one must go through. These community members are truly juvenile people, but they have found very satisfactory ways of life. The fact that such persons have been sadly distorted at a certain phase of their development and do not get anywhere near being an adult does not mean that they have become horribly abnormal and pass the rest of their lives in a mental hospital.

With regard to the patient's attitudes toward competition and compromise, since competition enjoys at least great tolerance, so the therapist can be quite direct in his questioning. Hence, one does no harm in asking the patient what *his* attitude toward competition is. On occasion he may ask, "What do you mean?" What does this amazing answer suggest? Is he puzzled about the meaning of *competition?* Then the interviewer may ask what puzzles the patient. If one accomplishes anything by such a question, then the interviewer proceeds: "What do you think of people who compromise?" Does he or would he compromise, never compromise, what could he compromise on, etc. And finally, what does he think of about those people who compromise?

At the same session, the therapist is alert at observing whether the interviewee is manifestly competitive. Has he got to know more about things than you do? Does he have to beat you to what you are driving at? On the other hand, a patient may turn out to be unduly conciliatory in an effort to give the therapist the feeling that he agrees with everything he says. The attitudes and utterances of the patient are quite significant. Unless the interviewer follows some sort of scheme for organizing his thoughts and procedure, he may overlook or misinterpret the patient's attitudes toward competition and compromise.

Space limitations do not permit the inclusion in a systematic fashion, of everything Sullivan wrote in *The Psychiatric Interview* (1954). With regard to *ambition*, it is frequently highly rewarded in a material sense. Sullivan wrote that it is worth noting that some people who strive "with tooth and nail" toward a certain type of goal are apt to have experienced astonishing successes and failures. It is said to be worthwhile also to notice not only how intense the ambition-driven person may be, but also the character of the goal he seeks. There are a few people who are intensely ambitious about one thing after another—depending on the situation they are in. Also, there are many other people, more significant because they are apt to hold important positions in society, who have been pursuing a more or less well-defined goal for years and years, doing everything short of homicide to get it. (Consider the Robber Barons.)

Initial schooling is frequently the period (the Juvenile Era) when the youngster gets an opportunity to correct the over-individualistic warp of acculturation which nearly everyone brings (or brought not long ago) to the school from the home. Initial schooling refers to the general period of grammar school. Until fairly recently, everyone attended. Secondly, it is in grammar school that one begins to learn social techniques to cover one's "real" feelings, and so, what happens thereafter is often not very revealing. Boys spend a lot of time playing baseball or football, and perhaps for an hour the girls are in the gym learning basketball. Sullivan wrote that the psychiatrist wants to know in general anything that will give him a notion of the way the patient felt toward grammar school. "Did he have a good time? Did he learn a lot? Did he like to learn the sort of things that were offered there? Does he have the impression that some teacher was wonderful to him?" In some ways, the boys' experiences in grammar school are a reflection of the happiness or unhappiness that they may have brought to school from home. (Parenthetically, Sullivan was dead when Soroken published his famous *The Sexual Revolution*.)

Sullivan did not follow a strict, orderly sequence as he prepared to inquire about the patient's experiences in college. If he had, he would unwittingly give the patient clues as to what security operations to use in order to defeat the purposes of the interview. This may happen because the self-system or anti-anxiety system is opposed to the therapist's efforts. No one wants to experience anxiety, despite his good intentions to get well. The interviewer, being thoroughly conscious of this phenomena, circumvents it by suddenly "leaping over high school to college." In this fashion, he can disturb the sets that are already beginning to develop—so the patient's attempts to adjust nicely to a certain type of questioning is thwarted. If the interviewer has already learned that the patient went to college, he may ask what the patient's experience there was. Did he fit in with the "studes," namely the very studious, or with the "socialites." Nowadays, one might ask if he fitted in with "the jocks." At any rate, it is better to be one or the other than the exception. It is better, in the United States, unless one really has a career spreading before him, to be a social success than a stude. "In other words, the American pattern of normality is to go to college and spend your parents' money, and to avoid any information that you can elude. . .So the interviewer wants to know where his patient stood in college" (Sullivan, 1956).

Interest in Boys' or Girls' Clubs

The psychiatrist will inquire if his patient, before he became a father, or before she became a mother, showed any particular interest in leading boys' clubs or girls' clubs, so that for years, he, or she, was a "big brother" or a "big sister." If the male patient did show such an interest in being a big brother, that is a fairly important clue to deficiencies in his preadolescence (Sullivan, 1956).

The Preadolescent Chum

Chumship was discussed in an earlier chapter, but we have to elucidate Sullivan's (1956) handling of chumship and any possible problems therein. He believed the preadolescent stage has so much to do with one's future social adaptability that not to have gotten some experience along the line of one's, at least potential, world of the future, seems very unfortunte. The patient is not conscious of any connection between an interest in boys' clubs and his relationship, if any, with his having a chum. The interviewer asks, "Does any stand out in your recolleciton as having been especially your chum in your early school years?" If the answer is yes, the interviewer will wish to learn what became of the friendship and of the friend. Are they great friends still? Further questioning as to what became of the chum will reveal the character of the relationship — if there was one. (The topic of the isolated boy is ignored in this chapter because it is not central to the topic under discussion — the quality of the chumship.) Further inquiry as to what became of the chum relationship is said to give the interviewer some notion as to its true character — whether it was an imaginary construct or an excerpt from actual life. If the patient has not thought of his chum for 20 years, he may become a bit surprised but is able to say, "Yes, I had a chum but I can't think of his name." After that, when the confirmation has been so strong, the therapist proceeds to a discussion of puberty.

PUBERTY

Sullivan (1956) often asked, "When did you undergo the pubertal change?" This question merely serves to introduce the topic, because most people do not know the time of its onset. Certain questions then follow as to when the patient's voice changed, when he began to shave, and when he had orgasm. In the case of a woman, the interviewer inquires when she first menstruated, when she noticed changes in the breasts, etc. Most people are pretty vague about such things. Yet, the patient may recall something important about one of them. If the pubertal change occurred two or three years late (in certain cultures it may arrive, in the instance of girls, at least two or three years earlier than the American norm — which for girls in those cultures is quite normal). If the patient is an American, and if the onset of puberty was very late, which is or may be very significant, he is likely to recall something about more than one thing related to puberty. This is vital in the sense that when puberty occurs two or three years after most of the people in the patient's group have undergone the change, this delay may be in itself a very serious warp in personality, and, in turn, foster further increasing problems. In the latter case, a great deal of misery in life is dated to the actual delay in puberty changes.

Once the interviewer has gone through the process of being *unable* to find out at what age a patient becomes pubescent, since most people forget, he is able to inquire somewhat further about those phenomena and he tries to find out whether there were any unfortunate ideas connected with them. For example, a woman may say, "I thought that something must have gone dreadfully wrong because I never dreamed of anyone bleeding there." This informs the interviewer that indeed there was unfortunate experience in the lady's background. In a "puritanical culture" things might have been worse. A long time ago, an elderly woman, who also thought that something was terribly wrong, because she never dreamed of anyone bleeding "there," and who was illiterate, revealed that when she first experienced such bleeding as a young girl she was horrified. Saying nothing to anyone, she fled down to a nearby river and waded in until she felt cleansed both morally and physically. All day long she sheltered in or near the river. In addition, her culture contained strict taboos about the mere mention of sexuality; so she was or felt trapped in what we call her biology—her culture, really.

Unfortunte Relationships in Early Adolescence

Having gone over all the amnesias, etc., of the puberty change, Sullivan would ask, "again rather categorically," "Is anyone recalled as having been a particularly bad influence in early adolescence?" If the answer is a hesitant "Yes," the therapist must use his judgement as to the degree of anxiety his patient may suffer from. The therapist must decide as to whether to proceed with the topic any further or postpone further questions to a time when they will be less risky and the patient is more secure. But, Sullivan would try not to forget the topic. If the unfortunate chum relationship has been treasured ever since it existed, that is significant. If the relationship has been "obliterated" as soon as possible, that sounds pretty healthy.

Sex Preference

Now that the interviewer has led the patient to thinking a little about or in terms of later adolescence, the former can ask whether he actually prefers men or women for companionship (Sullivan, 1956). If the patient is a woman, the inquiry is essentially similar. Should the patient manifest a little increase in reserve at this point, the interviewer can always modify his question "amiably" by saying "Well, it may vary with the moods that you're in. Of course you would prefer the company of women (or men if the patient is a woman) when you are retiring with a view to sexual satisfaction." When or if the patient looks suspiciously at the therapist, he was wrong, and that is revealing. The interviewer can continue smoothly by asking questions about whom the patient likes to dine with. Now that the topic of sexual preference has been brought out into the open, the interviewer can become specific. Sullivan would ask general questions often as a means of transition, to get a topic out in the open.

Use of Alcohol and Narcotics

The use of narcotics was widespread in the late nineteenth or early twentieth century and then, for a while, its use fell into abeyance. Sullivan (1956) asserted that a great many psychiatrists overlook the possibility of the use of narcotics which in his day, he said, was very much more restricted than the use of alcohol. His next statement has an almost poignant ring. "Don't utterly forget narcotics because you do not see a drug addict."

Sullivan would proceed to inquire about the patient's use of alcohol. He would ask when the patient was first drunk, with a "falling inflection," as if to apologize to the patient. Since nearly everyone has been drunk for a first time, so the patient would answer the query directly. But, it is more interesting to find out if the patient has been drunk a second time. Has he been fairly seriously injured when under the influence of alcohol, or more or less because he was intoxicated? A large proportion of people have been deterred "from going down the alcoholic road" by suffering some rather serious injury when they were drunk or when they were under a blending of dangerous activities, from which they had learned to use discretion. Then the interviewer wishes to know what the patient does when he takes quite a bit of liquor. "Does he become quarrelsome? Does he engage in a fight? Does he develop crying spells or weep easily? Or does he become very friendly with everyone?" The patient often answers this question by saying "I get sleepy"—not always a true statement. When the patient indicates that he shows a very disagreeable complex of behavior when drunk although he is not eager to talk about it, Sullivan does not question further on this topic. He knows or has learned that the behavior this patient has now revealed, is indicative of a very unhappy person who takes to alcohol when social pressure is too high and who, under the loss of inhibitions, reveals a good deal of the misery and hostility which have led him into grief with society. This misfortune is indicative that the personality is not well integrated, and has not achieved a high degree of development in late adolescence.

Sleep and Sleep Functions

The interviewer leads up gradually to sleep and sleep functions with some careful inquiry (Sullivan, 1956). Otherwise, if he does not, he will often "draw only misleading blanks." Most people have vague ideas about sleep and dreams—theirs. The interviewer may induce the topic by asking, "How much sleep do you seem to need?" The client may tell the therapist—and this is "well and good." If he does not, the therapist is at least "in the field" and can ask further questions. Is the patient a heavy or light sleeper? Then the interviewer wants to know if he ever dreams. If the patient is conscious of the fact that he dreams — some people believe they don't — he is queried as to whether he has nightmares. Sometimes, Sullivan said you come on a curious phenomenon. The person doesn't dream, but he has nightmares. This is a beautiful illustration of how the "same" words have different meanings to different people. And the psychiatrist must be eternally alert to that fact in therapy.

On occasion, when everything seems almost too normal, the therapist would indicate that he was not too pleased to discover that the patient sleeps eight hours every night, never dreams and never had a nightmare. Looking at the patient somewhat "irritably" the therapist asks "Did you ever have nightmares? Did anybody tell you about your having night terrors?" One who has known or seen those piercing blue eyes of Sullivan fixed on the patient like a laser beam, may seem sorry for "the victim." In fact, Sullivan was notoriously gentle with his patients, which for him was no mere procedure.

In any event, the patient's recollection gets stirred up sufficiently that he gives a sign of it, no matter what he wishes to conceal. It is reiterated that if he has had night terrors and has been a little upset by Sullivan's "irritation" and questioning, Sullivan would ask again what he dreams, when he dreams — despite the patient's denial of ever having dreams. If the patient persists in saying he never has dreams, Sullivan would abandon this line of questioning as a bad job. He would conclude that the patient has a very rigid self-organization, or he is a very guarded person who can still persist in his guardness despite any amount of pressure the therapist can safely apply.

The Sex Life

Sullivan (1956) emphatically rejects the notion that sex is in some curious fashion a mirror of personality. "Sex is important for the 20 minutes (some say 30 minutes) it may occupy from time to time that fills the rest of the time."

We have now reached the point when the interviewer may say to the patient: "Well, and what of the sex life? Are you very restrained in such things, or are you quite free? Are you promiscuous?" In response to the last question, the patient may stutter in response. Sullivan would continue to ask, "Well, how long has it been true? I don't suppose you've always been like that. Give me a history of your sexual experience. For example when did it begin" (Sullivan, 1956). Sullivan asserted that when the interviewer knows something about the beginning of the patient's developmental history he may know what is being discussed, but missing the beginning, he often just *thinks* he knows what is being discussed.

A remarkable number of people may recall their first encounter with another person. Although it may be a little hard to place in time, it is usually vividly registered in some way or other. But, if the patient's recall is skimpy, that is enough. The interviewer has gathered almost all the data he needs to guess about the patient's great problems and his probable adjustment to the set of circumstances that may be before him. After taking up a few more details, he stops his questions. All the things he discovered with his patient have much less to do with sex, than with personality as a whole. It is no secret that people often employ sexual behavior for prestige purposes, to avoid loneliness, to obtain money, popularity, or social status, as often seems the case with Hollywood figures, or the beautiful people. The sociological implication of the contemporary sexual culture is very suggestive but outside the scope of this book.

Courtships and Marriage

The social history, discussed previously, has already informed the interviewer of a good many things with respect to marriage, courtship, children, divorce.

Next comes an appraisal of interpersonal relations which characterize the marriage—its satisfactions and dissatisfactions, and the securities and insecurities which prevail. "I wish to know," Sullivan added, "whether the mate is the person who runs things, or is the person who is run, or whether husband and wife happily share in their dominance over each other." Who are the people outside the marriage (such as the patient's mother-in-law), that the mate is influenced by and particularly "never to be forgotten" neighbors. This is an indirect way of inquiring as to what extent is the mate harassed by a necessity of "keeping up with the Joneses." The interviewer has already inferred the sense of deep disappointment, if it exists, associated with the marriage relationship, not by asking.

Parenthood

Sullivan asked directly, "Is there a problem child in the family?" Should there be such, what is the explanation considered to be? Is there a preferred child, he needs to know, why is that child preferred? Has that preference any bad effects on that child, or any other child? In case it has, are there any neutralizing influences that can be learned from the client? The attitude of the parent-interviewee to school influences is said to be an excellent entering wedge, because school is "somewhat" impersonal partly because of the objectivity of the teacher, and partly because the youngster learns he is not the center of the universe — even if the mother believes he is. So, the child is compelled, unless he has already been severely undermined, to learn that he is one of many other children who are treated more or less alike. Social reality starts to bear on him. In addition to mother, are there relatives who may be influencing the client's child or children? There are two other things one must not forget to explore: whether the wife has had any miscarriages; and if some younger siblings died before the birth of the surviving child. If the client is the only surviving child, did the deaths of the other children, for example, increase his importance. The interviewer must also inquire about half-siblings because there may have been a divorce "on one side or the other," but also about wards or pseudosiblings in the family of approximately the same age who are looked after, since for some cause there is not adequate care anywhere else.

A vocational history as well as recreational history are important fields of data for assessment of personality with regard to the degree of maturity the client has achieved.

THE PERSONIFIED SELF

In an earlier chapter, it was pointed out the self can be distinguished as constituted by "good me" and "bad me" on the one hand, and the dissociated on the other. "Good me" and "bad me" tend to fuse to make up the self-system. The personified self is less inclusive than the self-system. The personified self is that part of the self-system which is reflected in statements about "I" or "Myself." As a rule, healthy people think of themselves as "good-me" but it is true that "bad-me" is also a part of the personified self, and in anxiety ridden people may predominate. But, the average healthy person has developed suave techniques for avoiding or minimizing anxiety-provoking situations, as well as employing various security operations which tend to bolster "good-me." Nevertheless, in an imperfect world, no one can avoid feeling "bad" at times. Strictly speaking, then, the personified self will usually protect and enhance the experience of "good-me" and the person will tend to think of himself as good. More exactly, the personified self is what the informant can tell about himself, or rather his self-system, as the content of the personified self.

Sullivan (1956) formulated a schematization of the personified self which is useful to the interviewer as he approaches the end of the Interview:

(1) What does the interviewee esteem and what does he disparage about himself ?

(2) To what experiences is the patient's self-esteem particularly unreasonably vulnerable?

(3) What are the characteristic "righting movements"—the security operations—which appear after the patient has been discomposed—made consciously anxious?

(4) How great are the interviewee's reserves of security? (a) For instance, how well is the patient's life justified? (This is a way of asking how well can the patient state characteristics of his life which are beyond doubt estimable and worthwhile) (b) Are there exalted purposes in his life which are demonstrated in action other than mere speech? (c) Are there secret sources of shame or enduring regret? (Witness Hawthorne's *The Scarlet Letter*) Should there be, what is the person's justification of his life?

While there are more questions the interviewer may ask, the following is revealing especially:

> How dearly does the interviewee actually value his life, and how steadfastly, and for how long has he so valued it?. . . What does the person consider to be worth more than himself? For what would he really sacrifice his life? When did he arrive at this conviction? How unalterable is it? (Sullivan, 1956)

The Termination of the Interview

In terminating the interview, the important thing is to consolidate whatever progress has been made (Sullivan, 1956). The consolidation of the interview's purpose is done by the following four steps: (1) the interviewer makes a *final statement* to the interviewee summarizing what he has learned during the course of the interview; (2) the interviewer gives the interviewee a *prescription of action* in which the interviewee is now to engage (for example, Sullivan had a female economist as a patient and advised her to resume a position as an economist instead of being a good housewife); (3) the interviewer makes a *final assessment* of the probable effects on the life course of the interviewee; and (4) there is the *formal leave-taking* between the interviewer and the interviewee.

Of course, the interviewer must give thought as to how the interviewee is going to take what he has been offered in this final interview.

No therapist, if he is conscientious, ever lets his patient go with a bleak, discouraging picture, in which the patient's self destruction would be the logical outcome. In short, there has to be the consolidation of some gain for the interviewee such that it points to a reasonably constructive picture for the patient's future. No matter what the condition of the patient, the therapist *never* offers a hopeless picture, even if there is one.

Sullivan quickly but gracefully accomplished the formal leave-taking — "There is no reason why one should have an exhausting turmoil in trying to say goodbye." The leave-taking should be a clean-cut respectful finish that does not confuse that which has been done (See Sullivan, 1956).

REFERENCES

Dewey, J. and Bentley, A.F. *Knowing and the Known*. The Beacon Press, Boston, 1949.

Einstein, A. and Infeld, L. *The Evolution of Physics*. Simon and Schuster, New York, 1938.

Havens, L.L. *Approaches to the Mind*. Little, Brown, and Co., Boston, 1973

Maxwell, C. Matter and motion, in Dewey, J. and Bentley, A.F. *Knowing and the Known*. The Beacon Press, Boston, 1949.

Sullivan, H.S. *The Interpersonal Theory of Psychiatry*. W.W. Norton, New York, 1953.

Sullivan, H.S. *The Psychiatric Interview*. W.W. Norton, New York, 1954.

Sullivan, H.S. *Clinical Studies in Psychiatry*. W.W. Norton, New York, 1956.

Index

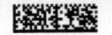